Clinical Radiology for Pediatricians

Dr Binit Sureka
MD (PGIMER, Chd.), DNB, MBA-HCA (FMS, Delhi)
MNAMS, Dip.Hosp. Admn.
Assistant Professor
Department of Radiology
Institute of Liver and Biliary Sciences (ILBS)
New Delhi

Dr Aliza Mittal
MBBS (Gold Medal), MD, DNB (Gold Medal), MNAMS
Dip. F. Med (CMC,Vellore)
Senior Resident
Department of Pediatrics
VMMC and Safdarjung Hospital
New Delhi

PEEPEE
PUBLISHERS AND DISTRIBUTORS (P) LTD.

Clinical Radiology for Pediatricians

Published by

Pawaninder P. Vij and Anupam Vij

Peepee Publishers and Distributors (P) Ltd.

Head Office: 160, Shakti Vihar, Pitam Pura,
Delhi-110 034 (India)

Correspondence Address:

7/31, First Floor, Ansari Road, Daryaganj
New Delhi-110 002 (India)

Ph: 65195868, 23246245, 9811156083

e-mail: peepee160@yahoo.co.in

e-mail: peepee160@rediffmail.com

e-mail: peepee160@gmail.com

www.peepeepub.com

First Edition: 2015

ISBN: 978-81-8445-177-1

To My Grandfather
Late Shree Balchand Sureka
and
To My Dadima...

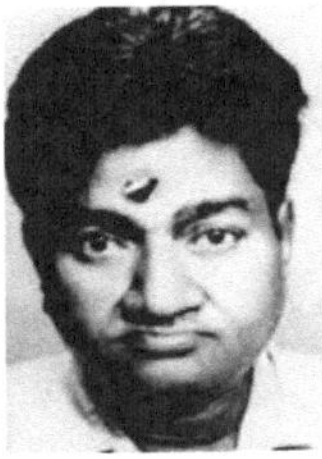 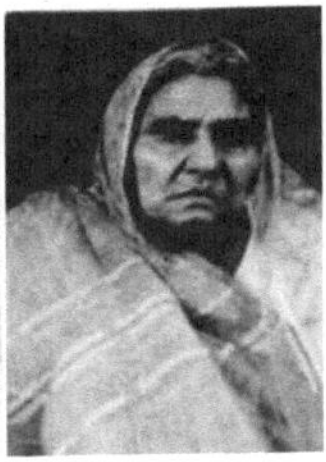

Foreword

Radiology has become an integral part of practical examinations for awarding professional degrees and diplomas in various specialties in India and abroad. Not only students, but our general practitioners should be well-informed about 'bread and butter' routine X-ray examinations, ultrasound and computed tomography (CT). Today, Radiology has become the key diagnostic tool for many diseases and has an important role in monitoring treatment and predicting outcome. Pediatric Radiology is a sub-specialisation developed to provide an integrated cohesive imaging service to the patients and their clinicians.

This book authored by Dr Sureka (Radiologist) and Dr Mittal (Pediatrician), whom I know personally are both young and dynamic academicians with keen interest in teaching and hence are also versed thoroughly with the problems faced by students appearing in the exams, and clinicians in everyday practice.

Dr Sureka did his Senior Residency at VMMC and Safdarjung Hospital, New Delhi. Dr Sureka has a brilliant and exceptional academic record and has attained postgraduate qualification in Radiology from prestigious Postgraduate Institute of Medical Education and Research (PGIMER), Chandigarh, India. He has also cleared DNB Radiology Exam of Diplomat of National Board of Examinations. In addition Binit has done Masters in Healthcare Administration (MBA–Healthcare) from Faculty of Management Studies, Delhi University, New Delhi and Diploma in Hospital Administration (PGDHA) from Apollo Hospitals, Hyderabad. He is an esteemed Member of National Academy of Medical Sciences. He has around 70 publications in various indexed and non-indexed national and international journals. This title would prove handy for the Pediatricians and Radiology trainee to overcome their fear of interpreting various Radiological signs and providing relevant differential diagnosis.

Dr Brij Bhushan Thukral
MD, FICR
Head of Department (Radiodiagnosis and Imaging)
Vardhman Mahavir Medical College and Safdarjung Hospital
New Delhi

Foreword

Knowledge of radiology in bedside clinics and patient management is as important as the clinical skills in today's scenario. Children are not merely little people or young adults, nor are the disorders to which they are susceptible, merely the variants of diseases in adults and hence the need for a text focusing particularly on Pediatric Radiology.

It is pertinent to know which essential radiological investigations should be done in a given clinical problem. It is very essential to maintain a balance in basic and advanced radiological investigations especially in market driven modern practices. This book tries to address few of these issues.

It has also been noticed that radiology is becoming an integral part of not only bedside patient care, but also carries a lot of marks in various medical exams in Pediatrics such as MBBS, MD and DNB.

This title concisely covers all aspects of Radiology one requires to know in day-to-day practice along with all important questions pertaining to Radiology asked in exams. I'm sure students appearing in these exams would find it handy and as useful as the clinicians as a pocket guide to bedside Radiology.

The book has been authored by Dr Aliza Mittal and Dr Binit Sureka, both of whom are young, dynamic, toppers in academics and are always striving for excellence.

Dr Aliza Mittal, has been associated with our department for past many years. She is a young and dynamic pediatrician who has always been an asset to our department. Having herself appeared for and cleared MD and DNB exams and keen on teaching the postgraduates. She is well versed with the problems faced by students in answering the Radiology based questions, which have been adequately covered in the text. I'm sure this book would be a good help for such students.

I hereby wish good luck to both the authors.

Dr KC Aggarwal
MD
Head of Department, Department of Pediatrics
Vardhman Mahavir Medical College and Safdarjung Hospital
New Delhi

Preface

Knowledge on its own is nothing, but the application of useful knowledge, now that is powerful. Nearly 100 years from its birth, radiology continues to grow as though still in its adolescence. Radiology has evolved from purely diagnostic devices to interventional technologies. Today Radiology is a key part of clinical practice across a wide range of medical disciplines. It is usually the best, minimally invasive way of diagnosing, treating or monitoring disease and injury.

Radiology has become an integral part of any exam whether in India or abroad. This short book illustrates common entities encountered in day-to-day Pediatric practice. This work is done keeping in mind needs of Pediatricians – residents, students, consultants and teachers in medical colleges. It would come handy for students appearing in various exams such as DNB-OSCE, MRCPCH and MD exams. This book contains basics like sequential interpretation of chest and abdominal radiographs. Images of common entities, differential diagnosis and various signs in Radiology are briefly discussed in this handbook.

I earnestly hope this book will enlighten the Pediatricians in clinical practice with additional knowledge and expertise and help them improve their Radiological skills.

Binit Sureka
Aliza Mittal

Acknowledgements

This book is an example of dreams turning into reality and it wouldn't have been possible without the blessings of our grandparents.

I am thankful to God for giving me opportunity to learn Radiology from PGIMER, Chandigarh. I am fortunate to have stalwarts like Professor N Khandelwal (HOD Radiodiagnosis, PGIMER, Chandigarh), Dr Akshay Saxena, Dr Kushaljit S Sodhi as my teachers. Their keen interest in teaching Radiology and academic environment of the Institute motivated me to contribute to the society.

We are also thankful to Dr KC Aggarwal (HOD Pediatrics, VMMC and Safdarjung Hospital) and Dr Harish Chellani for always being a guiding force and a constant source of inspiration.

My earnest thanks to Dr BB Thukral (HOD Radiology, VMMC and Safdarjung Hospital), Dr MK Mittal and Dr Yatish Aggarwal who constantly motivated me in research and writing.

I wish to express my gratitude to my colleagues Dr Kalpana and Dr Ankur in giving valuable inputs.

Words cannot express our thankfulness to our parents, family and friends for constantly supporting and encouraging us.

...And why of all the attitudes you can acquire, it's the attitude of gratitude that can be the most important and life-changing.

Binit Sureka
Aliza Mittal

Contents

References and Suggested Readings

1. *Caffey's Pediatric Diagnostic Imaging.*

2. *Diagnostic Radiology Pediatric Imaging (AIIMS-MAMC-PGI Imaging Series).*

3. *Radiology Review Manual (Dahnert, Radiology Review Manual).*

4. *Textbook of Radiology and Imaging by David Sutton.*

5. *Essentials of Pediatric Radiology: A Multimodality Approach (Cambridge Medicine).*

6. *Aids to Radiological Differential Diagnosis. Stephen Chapman, Richard Nakielny.*

1

Chapter

Introduction

TECHNICAL ASPECTS IN CHEST X-RAY

1. **Rotation:** In a properly centred film, the medial ends of the clavicles should be equidistant from the vertebral spinous processes at D4/D5 level. A rotated film is not properly centred film and the lung area nearest to the film appears less translucent.
2. **Penetration:** In an adequately penetrated film, the vertebral bodies and disc spaces should be just visible up till D8/D9 level. In an over penetrated film, all thoracic vertebrae are visible behind the heart shadow and lungs appear darker. In an under penetrated film, no vertebrae are visible.
3. **Degree of Inspiration:** When anterior ends of the sixth ribs or posterior ends of the tenth rib are above the right hemi diaphragm, it is said to be adequate.

   On an expiratory film, the heart shadow appears larger and there is crowding of bronchovascular markings in the basal regions.
4. **Artefacts:** Radiographic artefacts due to techniques, hair artefacts, external medical devices, nasogastric tubes, clothes, etc.

Difference Between Chest PA and AP View:

PA view	AP view
Standard view, ambulatory patient, older children	Done for patients unable to stand, portable radiographs, neonates and small children
Scapula away from the lung fields	Scapulae overlies the lung fields
Clavicles away from the apices	Clavicles projected over the apices
Neural arches clearly seen	Disc spaces clearly seen
No magnification effect	Superior mediastinum and heart appears enlarged due to magnification factor
Ribs oriented obliquely	Ribs more horizontal
Good quality	Lower quality

Different Views in Chest X-Rays and their Significance:

Chest View	Clinical Importance
PA	Standard view
AP	For portable, ICU, neonates and small children
Lateral	Hidden areas of lung
Apicogram	Apical region
Lordotic	Middle lobe
Decubitus	Small pleural effusion and small pneumothorax
Oblique	Retrocardiac area, chest wall, posterior CP angles
Expiratory view	Pneumothorax
Penetrated view	Left lower lobe and cardiac chamber visualization

Hidden Areas of Lung in a Chest X-Ray:

1. The apical regions.
2. Mediastinum and hila.
3. Retrodiaphragmatic area.
4. Lung behind bones.

Interpretation of Chest X-Ray:

1. First look at name, age, sex of patient if provided in the film. Also try to seek some clinical information before interpreting.
2. Then check the technical aspects.
3. Costophrenic and cardiophrenic angles.
4. Cardiac size, borders and mediastinum.
5. Lung parenchyma.
6. Hila.
7. Trachea.
8. Diaphragms – also try to look below the diaphragms for stomach bubble, gas shadows and calcification if any.
9. Hidden areas.
10. Soft tissues.
11. Bones.
12. Four corners of the film.

SEGMENTAL ANATOMY OF LUNG

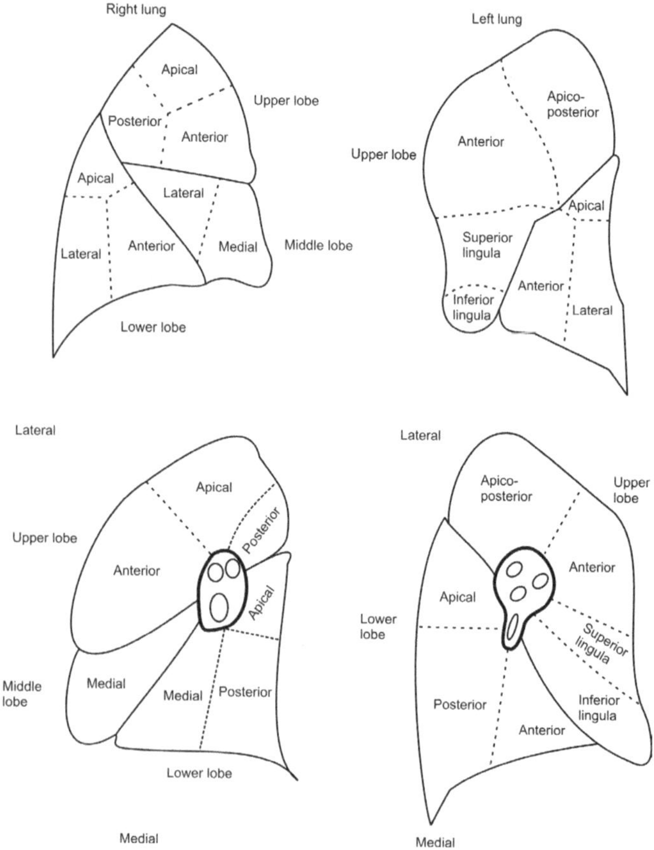

Figure 1.1

Effective Radiation Doses in Various Procedures

Procedure	Radiation dose in millisievert (mSv)
Chest X-ray (PA view)	0.02
CT chest	7
CT chest low dose	1.5
IVP	3
CT abdomen and pelvis	10
Skull X-ray	0.1
NCCT head	2
NCCT head plain and with contrast	4
X-ray spine	1.5
X-ray limbs and joints	0.06
Bone densitometry (DEXA)	0.001
Barium swallow	1.5
Barium meal	3
Barium meal follow through	3
Barium enema	7

Guidelines for Contrast Imaging

Nil Per Oral Guidelines for Contrast CT and MRI

Age	Solids and Milk/ Formula	Clear liquids
> 3 years	Stop 6-8 hours before sedation	Stop 2-3 hours before sedation
6 months – 3 years	Stop 6 hours before sedation	Stop 2-3 hours before sedation
< 6 months	Stop 4-6 hours before sedation	Stop 2 hours before sedation

2
Chapter

Chest

HYALINE MEMBRANE DISEASE (RESPIRATORY DISTRESS SYNDROME)

May be suspected in the setting of a preterm newborn who presents with respiratory distress. The baby may or may not have received antenatal steroids. It occurs as a result of progressive atelectasis of the alveoli due to deficiency of the lung surfactant.The child may be asymptomatic initially and the complete picture may take 6-12 hours to develop. The baby may have tachypnoea with prominent grunting, severe subcostal and intercostal indrawing, nasal flaring and cyanosis. The breath sounds may be normal or diminished with harsh tubular quality.

Findings on Chest X-Ray:

The X-Rays depend on the severity of the disorder with poorly inflated lungs being the cardinal feature.

Grading of HMD

Grade 1–Initially the radiographs may look normal or show minimal granular pattern or fine homogenous ground glass shadowing.

Grade 2–When disease becomes more severe, the granular densities become more apparent and represent overlapping collapsed areas, and widespread air bronchogram may become visible.

Grade 3–Consists of confluent alveolar shadowing.

Grade 4–Complete white out of the lung fields which will obscure the cardiac border in more severe cases.

Complications: Pulmonary interstitial emphysema (linear lucencies 1-4 mm radiating outwards from the hilum up to the periphery of lungs), pneumothorax, pneumomediastinum.

Ultrasound: Increased retrodiaphragmatic hyperechogenicity.

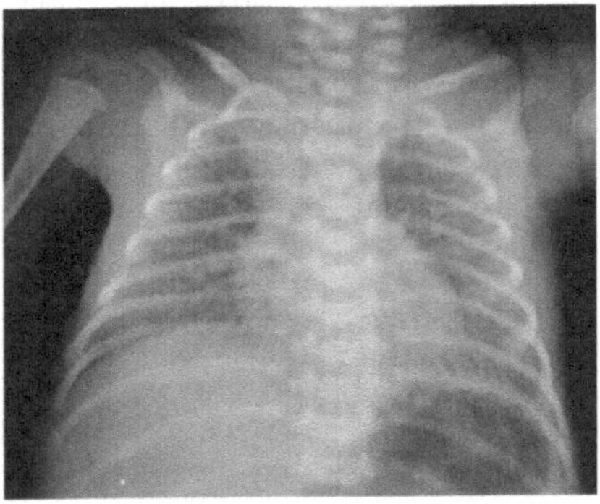

Figure 2.1: Chest radiograph showing Stage 2 HMD with granular opacities in bilateral lungs

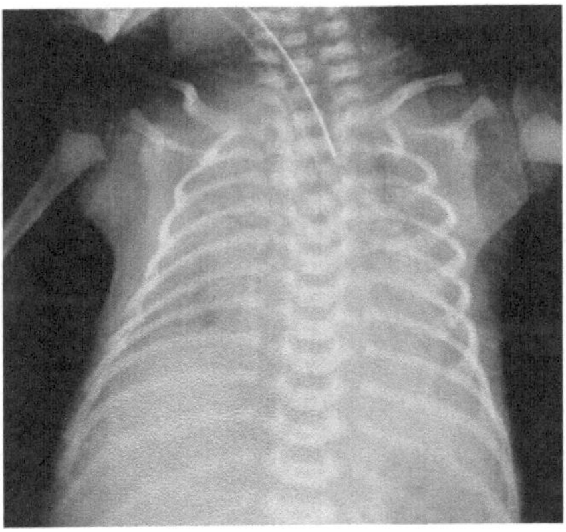

Figure 2.2: Chest radiograph showing Stage 4 HMD with complete white out lungs with endotracheal tube *in situ*

MECONIUM ASPIRATION SYNDROME

Usually seen in babies born through meconium stained liquor when thick particulate meconium gets aspirated into the lungs with the first breath. Clinical presentation may vary from persistent tachypnoea to severe respiratory distress. An increased anteroposterior chest diameter may be seen along with grunting and severe subcostal and intercostal retractions, cyanosis and may complicate into airblock syndromes. It may resolve by 72 hours or may require assisted ventilation with a high risk of mortality.

Findings on Chest X-Ray:

Findings on chest radiograph are variable. Generalised hyperinflated lungs may be seen due to incomplete bronchial obstruction. Nodular opacities may be seen due to atelectasis, chemical pneumonitis or pneumonia.

Complications: Pneumothorax, pneumomediastinum, pulmonary edema, pulmonary hemorrhage, persistent pulmonary hypertension.

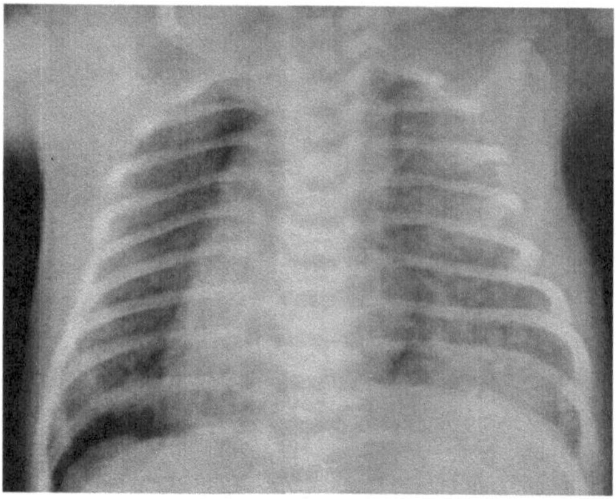

Figure 2.3: Chest radiograph showing mildly hyperinflated lungs with nodular opacities in bilateral lungs in a case of meconium aspiration syndrome

TRANSIENT TACHYPNOEA OF THE NEWBORN

Usually follows an uneventful delivery of a term or preterm baby either through vaginal route or by caesarean section, but more often in term babies born by caesarean section. Characterized by tachypnea or sometimes even retractions and expiratory grunting and cyanosis. Most infants recover rapidly within 3 days.

Findings on Chest X-Ray:

Normal to mild overinflated lungs, mild cardiomegaly, minimal effusion (fluid in minor fissure), and perihilar infiltrates.

May show reticulonodular pattern of HMD (lungs in HMD appear under aerated while in TTN appears normal to mildly over inflated). Chest radiograph may mimic meconium aspiration syndrome.

Ultrasound: Difference in lung echogenicity between upper and lower lung zones.

"Double lung point sign" – Compact comet-tail artifacts in lower lung zones.

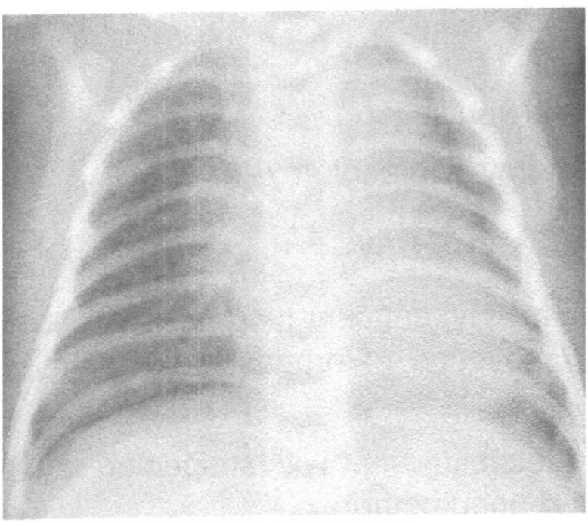

Figure 2.4: Chest radiograph in a newborn showing mildly overinflated lungs with perihilar infiltrates in a case of transient tachypnea of newborn

PNEUMOTHORAX

Presents with abrupt onset of dyspnoea, cyanosis and chest pain. Severity of symptoms depend on the extent of lung collapse and the amount of pre-existing lung disease. Usually it presents with tachypnea, retractions and diminished or absent breath sounds with a hyper-resonant percussion note over the hemithorax. Mediastinal shift may be noted. When fluid is also present there is an area of sharp demarcation between the flat note of percussion overlaying the fluid and the tympanic percussion note over the pneumothorax.

Causes of Pneumothorax

Primary Idiopathic.

Secondary to:

- Congenital lung malformations.
- Asthma.
- Airblock syndromes.
- Infections–pneumonias/lung abscess.
- Diffuse lung disease-Marfan's, Ehler-Danlos syndrome.
- Trauma.
- Mechanical ventilation.
- Tracheostomy/Thoracotomy.

Findings on Chest X-Ray:

Upright patient: Hyperlucent lung; visible visceral pleural line confirmed by absence of bronchovascular markings supero-lateral to this line.

Expiratory or decubitus view with suspected side up may help in detecting small pneumothorax.

Tension pneumothorax: Shift of the mediastinum and inversion of hemidiaphragm.

Supine patient: Strong clinical suspicion, relative lucency of lungs. In addition two important signs may be seen.

"Deep sulcus sign" – CP angle appears abnormally deep and lucent.

"Double diaphragm sign" – Visualization of anterior CP angle as an edge separate from diaphragm.

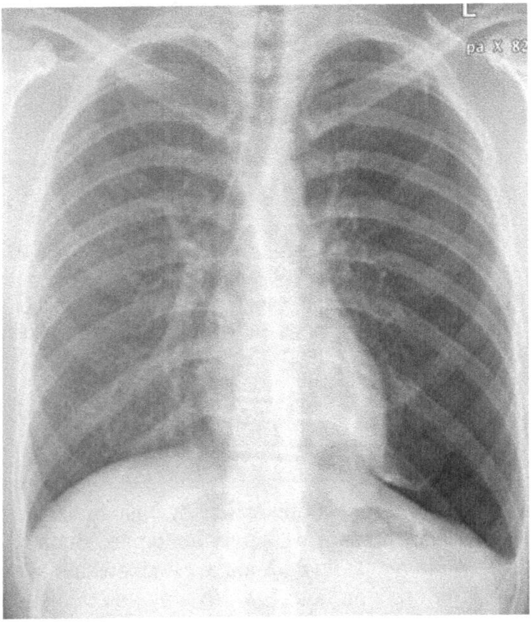

Figure 2.5: Chest radiograph showing left lucent hemithorax with absent bronchovascular markings and mild mediastinal shift to the contralateral side suggestive of pneumothorax

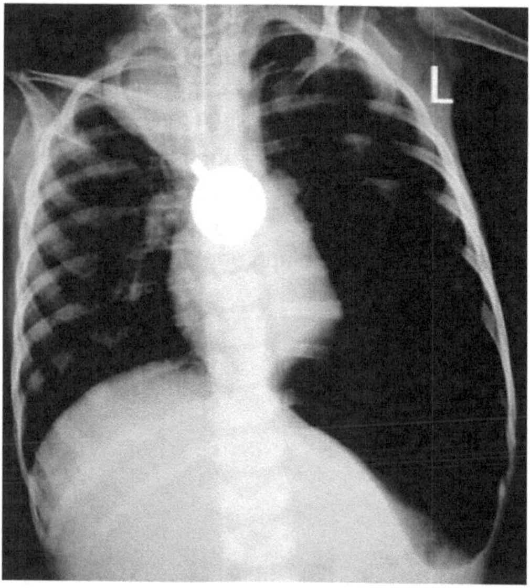

Figure 2.6: Chest radiograph showing left lucent hemithorax with absent bronchovascular markings and inversion of left hemidiaphragm in a case of tension pneumothorax. Note is made of endotracheal tube and a metallic artefact in midline

PNEUMOMEDIASTINUM

It presents as transient stabbing chest pain radiating to the neck. It may also present with pain abdomen. Subcutaneous emphysema is a cardinal feature. A mediastinal crunch "Hamman Sign" may be heard, which may be confused with a friction rub. Cardiac dullness to percussion may be reduced.

Causes

- Chronic pulmonary diseases.

- After adenotonsillectomy and dental extraction.
- Penetrating trauma.
- Diabetic ketoacidosis.
- Acute gastroenteritis.
- Inhaled foreign body.
- Acute severe asthma is the most common cause of Pneumomediastinum in older children and adolescents.

Findings on Chest X-Ray:

Spinnaker sail sign – Elevation of the thymus.

Double bronchial wall sign – Visualization of both sides of bronchial wall.

Continuous diaphragm sign –Visualization of entire diaphragm.

Tubular artery sign – Air outlining the aorta.

Ring around artery sign – Air outlining the pulmonary artery.

Pneumomediastinum	Pneumothorax	Pneumopericardium
Appears linear	Crescent shaped	Ovoid in shape
Air extends above level of aortic arch	No such extension	Does not extend above aortic arch
Pericardium not seen	Pericardium not seen	Pericardium may be visualized
Visualization of septae	Septae not visualized	Septae not visualized
Decubitus view shows no shift of mediastinal air	Shift of air present	Shift of air present
Air may dissect into neck, soft tissues	Usually absent	Usually absent

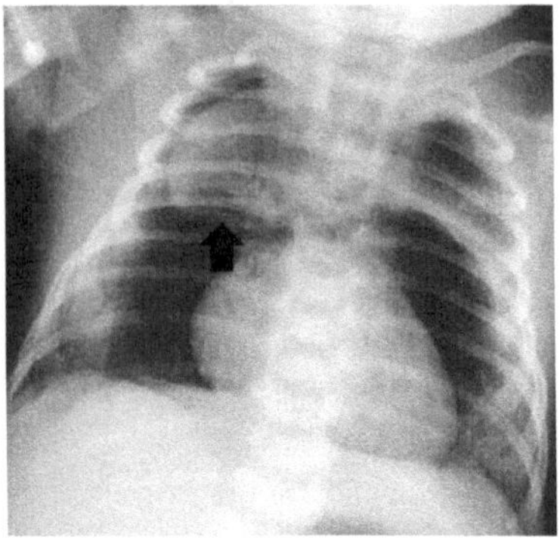

Figure 2.7: Chest radiograph showing elevated thymus (arrow) in a case of pneumomediastinum

PLEURAL EFFUSION

Findings on Chest X-Ray:

Upright patient: Homogenous opacity in lower chest with obliteration of CP angle and hemidiaphragm. Upper margin is concave and higher laterally. Mediastinal shift may or may not be seen depending upon the amount of pleural fluid. The highest lateral margin of haziness or 'meniscus' reflects the true level of pleural fluid. Absence of mediastinal shift in presence of large effusion should strongly suggest malignant etiology.

Blunting of CP angle – 175 ml.

Lateral decubitus film – 10 ml.

Supine patient: Hazy veil like opacity, absent air bronchogram and preserved bronchovascular markings.

Subpulmonic effusion: High hemidiaphragm with contour showing lateral peak. On the left side, distance of more than 2 cm from lung base to top of stomach bubble is suggestive. Subpulmonic effusion are mobile and changes with posture.

Lamellar effusion: Fluid accumulation between lung and visceral pleura seen in heart failure. On X-ray seen as a vertical band of soft tissue between lung and chest wall; is fixed and does not change with posture.

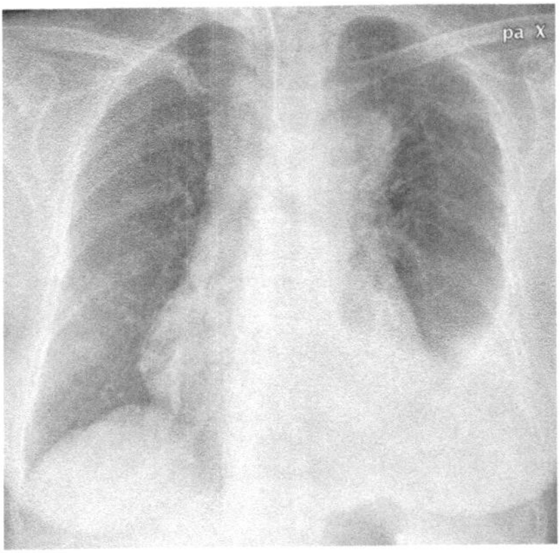

Figure 2.8: Chest radiograph showing homogenous opacity in left hemithorax with obscuration of left hemidiaphragm and raised lateral margin suggestive of left pleural effusion

BULLAE

Findings on Chest X-Ray:

Chest radiograph shows focal area of lucent lung field with absent bronchovascular markings. Bullae are rounded, inner margins appear concave relative to the chest wall, do not conform to the costophrenic angle when present at the lung base while pneumothorax is typically crescent shaped, inner margins are convex relative to chest wall (due to visceral pleural line) and tapers towards the lung base.

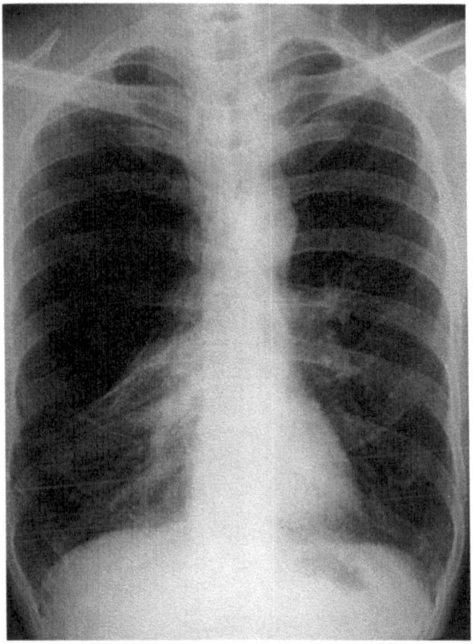

Figure 2.9: Chest radiograph showing oval shaped cystic lesion in right lung with absent bronchovascular markings and inner margins concave relative to chest wall suggestive of bulla

CONGENITAL LOBAR EMPHYSEMA (CLE)

Findings on Chest X-Ray:

Lung involvement: Most common in left upper lobe followed by right middle lobe and right upper lobe. CT scan is diagnostic.

Chest radiograph shows hyperinflated lung lobe with splaying and stretching of bronchovascular markings, atelectasis of adjacent lobe and evidence of contralateral mediastinal shift.

DD is pneumothorax which shows absence of bronchovascular markings.

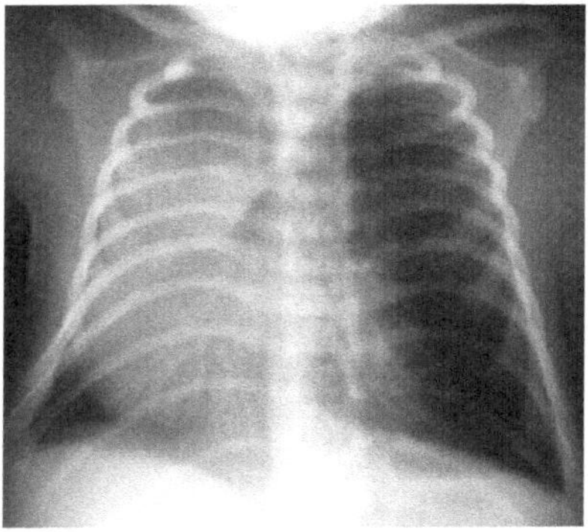

Figure 2.10: Chest radiograph showing relatively lucent left lung with stretched bronchovascular markings and contralateral mediastinal shift in a case of congenital lobar emphysema

CONGENITAL PULMONARY AIRWAY MALFORMATION (CPAM)

Previously called as congenital cystic adenomatoid malformation (CCAM).

Findings on Chest X-Ray:

Unilateral involvement usually seen.

Type I: Most common; multiple or single large cysts which communicate with the bronchial tree.

Type II: Multiple cysts 0.5-1.2 cm which communicate with the bronchial tree.

Type III: Least common; multiple small <0.5 cm cysts and may appear solid on imaging.

Differential Diagnosis:

CLE, congenital diaphragmatic hernia, pneumatoceles, mesenchymal cystic hamartoma, bronchogenic cyst.

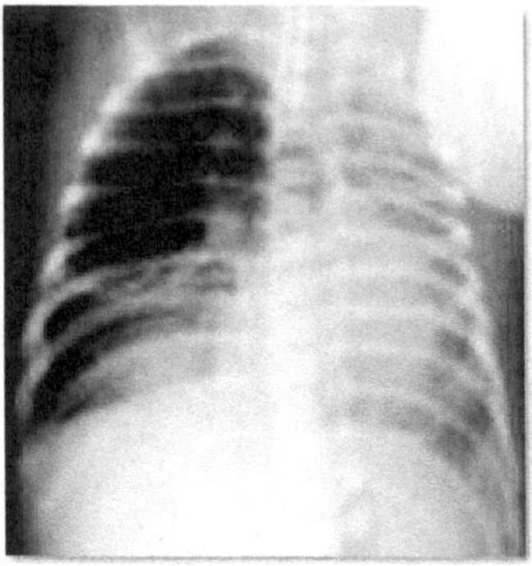

Figure 2.11: Chest radiograph showing cystic lesions in right upper and mid zone with absent bronchovascular markings

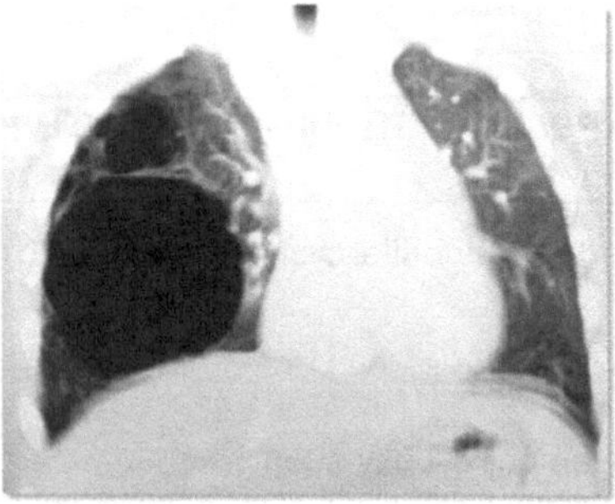

Figure 2.12: Coronal reformatted CT scan image showing multiple cysts in right lung in a case of CCAM

CONGENITAL DIAPHRAGMATIC HERNIA (CDH)

Findings on Chest X-Ray:

Location may be anterolateral (Morgagni hernia); posterolateral (Bochdalek hernia); or in the central tendon of diaphragm.

Chest radiograph findings depends upon the content of herniated bowel. Initially, when the bowel loops are fluid filled, opacity is seen in the affected side with contralateral mediastinal shift. As the air distends the bowel loops characteristic bowel signature may be seen in the thorax with paucity of bowel loops in the abdomen and non-visualized hemidiaphragm.

Ultrasound, CT or a contrast study of the GIT may be helpful.

Differential Diagnosis:

CCAM, CLE (infected), pneumatoceles, mesenchymal cystic hamartoma.

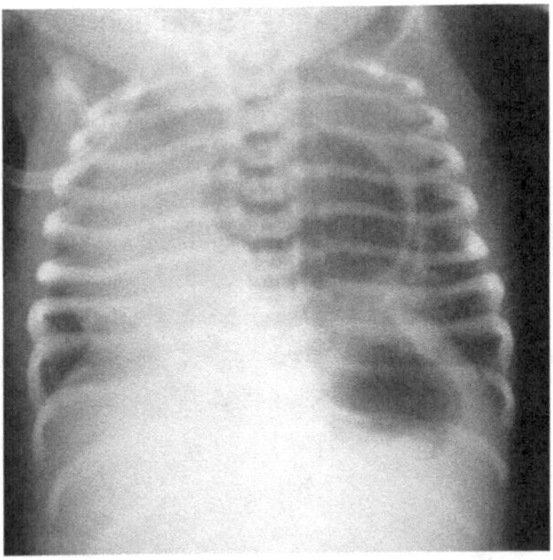

Figure 2.13: Chest radiograph showing bowel loops in left hemithorax with non-visualized left hemidiaphragm in a case of congenital diaphragmatic hernia

EVENTRATION OF DIAPHRAGM

Diaphragmatic eventration refers to an abnormal contour of the diaphragmatic dome due to congenitally thin muscular portion of hemidiaphragm. Over time this region stretches and on inspiration does not contract normally.

More commonly, it is seen on right side near the anteromedial portion of the right hemidiaphragm. When it involves the left side, usually whole of left hemidiaphragm is involved.

Findings on Chest X-Ray:

Seen as a smooth hump on the normal contour of the hemidiaphragm.

Differential Diagnosis:

Lung pathologies – Consolidation, mass, infarction, collapse.

Pleural pathologies – Mass, subpulmonic effusion.

Diaphragmatic pathologies – Subdiaphragmatic collection, phrenic nerve palsy, hemiplegia.

Rarely liver, splenic, colonic and stomach masses.

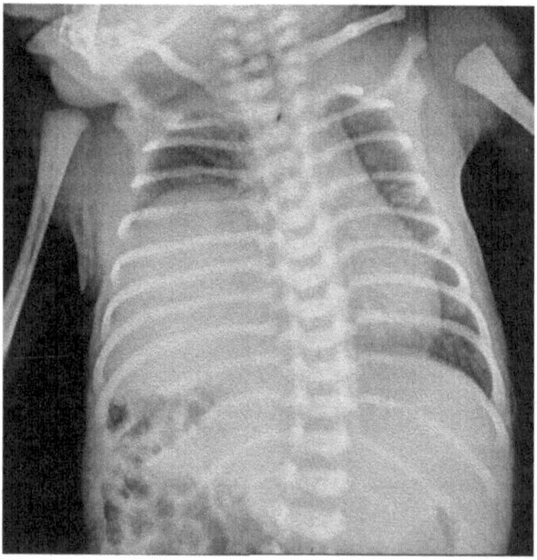

Figure 2.14: Chest radiograph showing homogenous opacity in right mid and lower zone with non-visualized right hemidiaphragm and mild mediastinal shift to the left side in a surgically proven case of eventration of diaphragm

PULMONARY THROMBOEMBOLISM

Findings on Chest X-Ray:

Earliest finding is small pleural effusion. Hampton's hump – peripheral wedge shaped consolidation; raised ipsilateral hemidiaphragm; plate-like atelectasis; Westermark sign – oligemia of lungs; Fleischner sign – prominent central pulmonary artery.

CT pulmonary angiography is diagnostic.

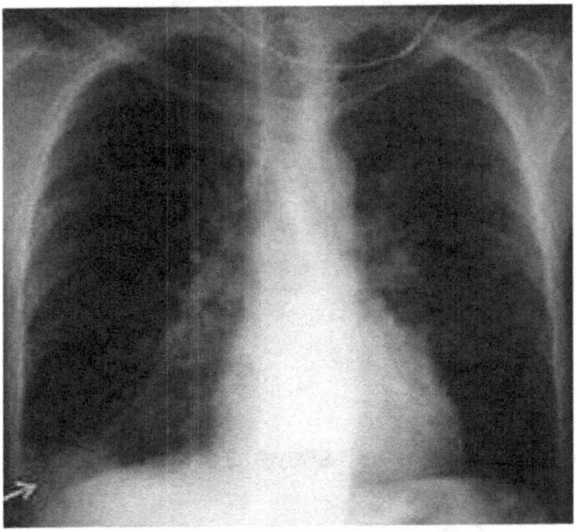

Figure 2.15: Chest radiograph showing a peripheral wedge-shaped opacity (arrow) suggestive of pulmonary infarct and prominent bronchovascular markings in right lower zone in a proven case of pulmonary thromboembolism

BRONCHIECTASIS

Findings on Chest X-Ray:

Multiple cystic, ring shadow (bronchus seen end on) or tram-like lucencies (parallel course of bronchial walls), bronchial wall thickening. In case of secondary infection mucous plugging, air-fluid levels may be seen.

HRCT chest is diagnostic. Inner luminal diameter of bronchus exceeds the diameter of adjacent pulmonary artery, lack of normal tapering of bronchus, signet ring sign–denoted by artery resembling a jewel abutting the dilated bronchus which appears as a ring.

Most common cause of bronchiectasis is post infectious.

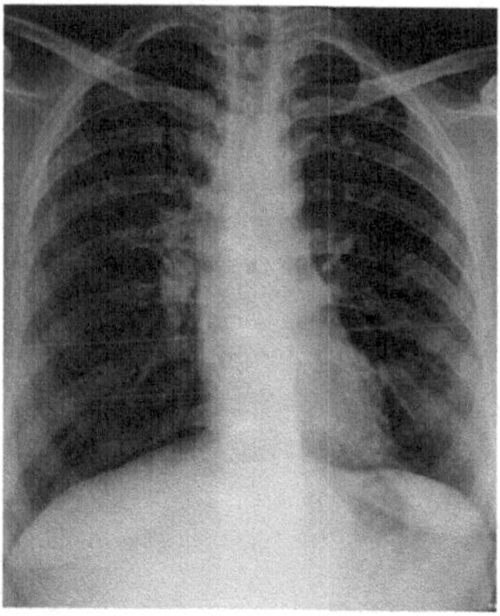

Figure 2.16: Chest radiograph showing cystic bronchiectasis in bilateral lungs

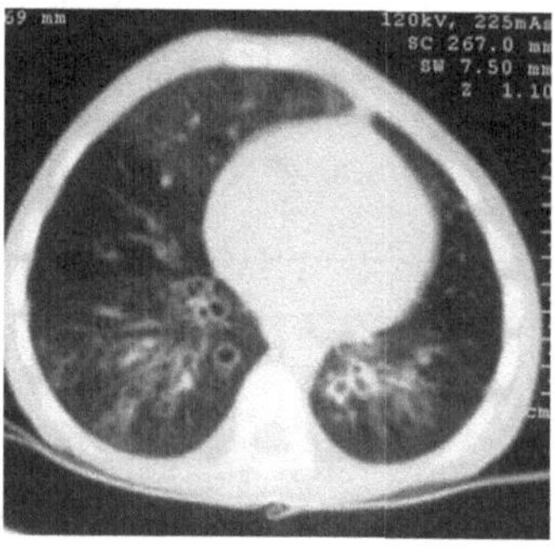

Figure 2.17: Axial Chest CT scan image showing cystic bronchiectatic changes in bilateral lower lobes

ASTHMA

Findings on Chest X-Ray:

Chest radiographs are usually normal. Occasionally, one may find hyperlucency of lung fields, bronchial wall thickening or complications like allergic bronchopulmonary aspergillosis, lobar collapse, atelectasis, pneumonia, pneumomediastinum, pneumothorax, pulmonary interstitial emphysema, and subcutaneous emphysema.

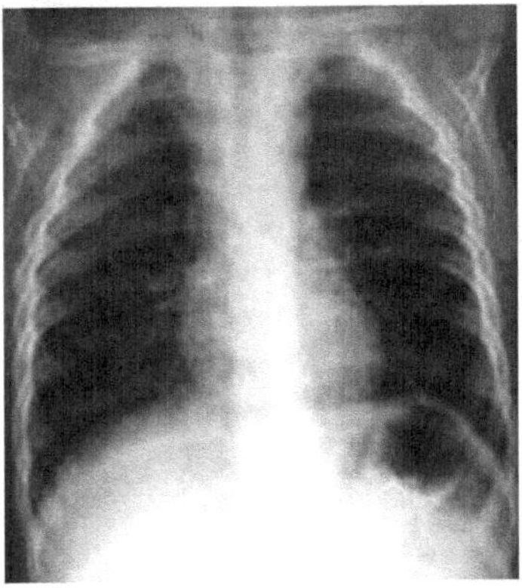

Figure 2.18: Chest radiograph showing hyperlucency in bilateral lungs in a case of asthma (*Note:* DD in a child is foreign body aspiration)

PERICARDIAL EFFUSION

Findings on Chest X-Ray:

Findings seen when fluid is more than 250 ml.

"Water bottle configuration of the heart" due to symmetrical enlargement of cardiac silhouette; pencil sharp outline of heart borders due to diminished cardiac pulsations; rapidly appearing cardiomegaly; loss of retrosternal clear space on lateral radiograph.

Other signs that may be seen are "fat-pad sign" – separation of epicardial from retrosternal fat >2 mm and "differential density sign" – increased lucency at heart borders due to density difference between fluid and myocardium.

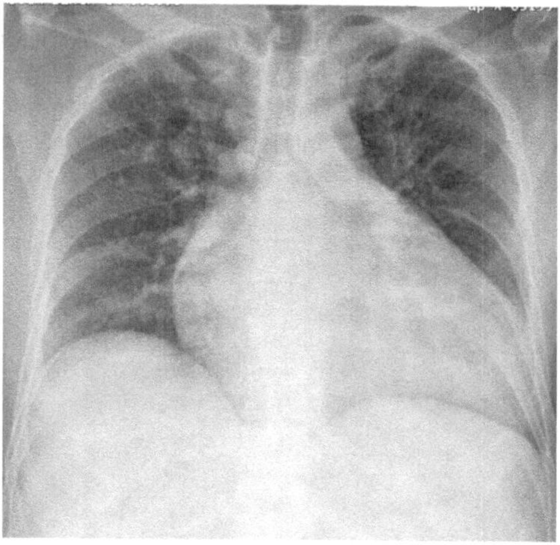

Figure 2.19: Chest radiograph showing globular heart with narrow pedicle in a case of pericardial effusion

LUNG ABSCESS

Findings on Chest X-Ray:

Chest radiograph findings depends upon the stage and contents of abscess. Acute lung abscess is seen as an area of ill-defined opacity with surrounding consolidation. Later, when there is communication with the bronchus, air-fluid levels are seen and the walls appear thick and shaggy.

Contrast-enhanced CT or sometimes ultrasound of the chest when the abscess is located peripherally is diagnostic.

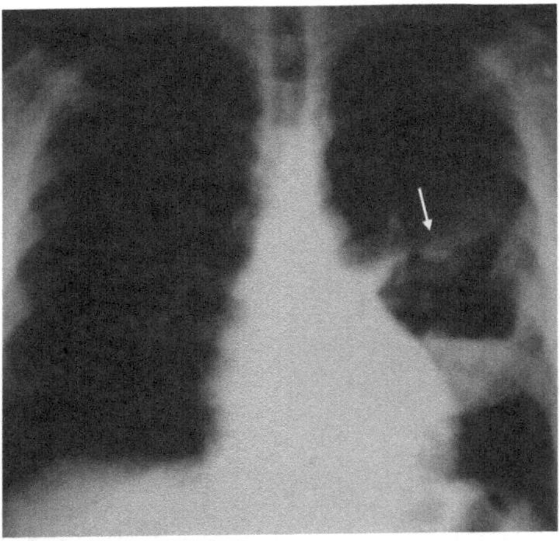

Figure 2.20: Chest radiograph showing thick-irregular walled cavitating lesion (arrow) in left mid and lower zone with fluid level suggestive of lung abscess

NORMAL THYMUS

Findings on Chest X-Ray:

On chest radiograph, normal thymus is seen as a triangular sail-shaped structure in superior mediastinum. The thymus has well defined borders and may project to one or both the sides of the mediastinum. The borders may be wavy in outline due to indentation by the costal cartilages which is also known as "wave sign of Mulvey" or "thymic wave sign".

The normal thymus has a well-defined sharp vertical lateral border, and forms a notch with the heart border which differentiates it from right upper lobe consolidation. Also it shrinks in size on deep inspiration.

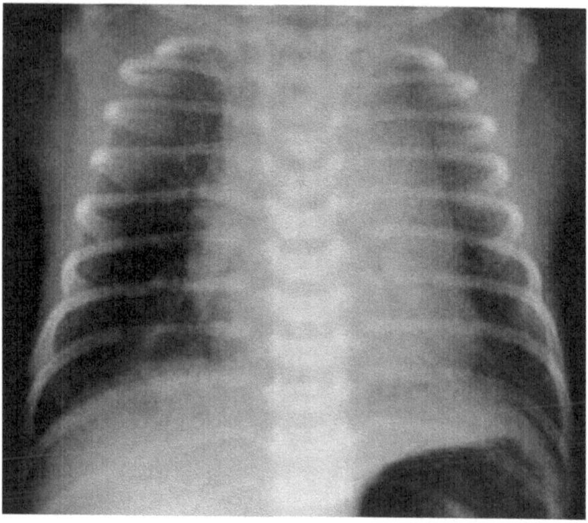

Figure 2.21: Chest radiograph showing normal cardiothymic shadow in a newborn

MILIARY TUBERCULOSIS

Findings on Chest X-Ray:

Small discrete nodules 2-4 mm in diameter (Millet-seed sized) scattered in bilateral lung parenchyma.

Differential Diagnosis:

Infections–Tuberculosis, fungal, chickenpox; Metastases; Haemosiderosis secondary to mitral stenosis; sarcoidosis; HMD; Histiocytosis X; amyloidosis; secondary hyperparathyroidism; alveolar microlithiasis and occupational lung diseases (seen in adults).

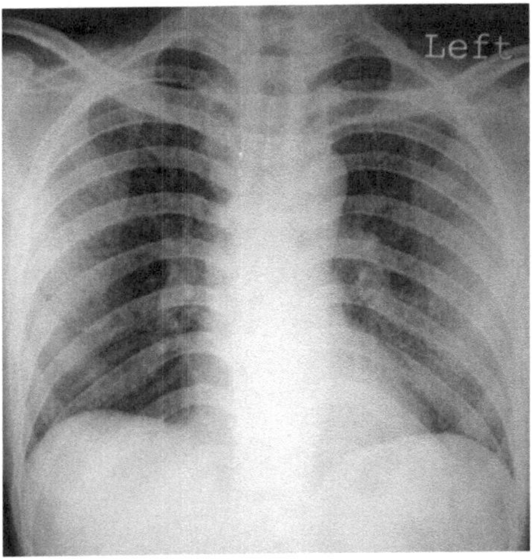

Figure 2.22: Chest radiograph showing small nodules in bilateral lungs suggestive of miliary tuberculosis.

PULMONARY EDEMA

Findings on Chest X-Ray:

Radiographic findings of interstitial edema precedes airspace involvement. Interstitial edema is seen as Kerley B lines (thickening of interlobular septa). Kerley B lines are 1-2 mm wide and 3-6 cm in length seen in sub-pleural location perpendicular to the pleura. Other findings are peribronchial cuffing (thickened walls of airway), perihilar haziness. Occasionally lamellar effusion may be seen.

Alveolar edema is seen as airspace opacities involving the central lung producing 'bat's wing' pattern.

Cardiogenic pulmonary edema is characterized by central distribution, upper lobe blood diversion, broad vascular pedicle, pleural effusion, cardiomegaly, peribronchial cuffing, dilated azygous vein while non-cardiogenic pulmonary edema is seen as patch peripheral involvement with normal width of the vascular pedicle.

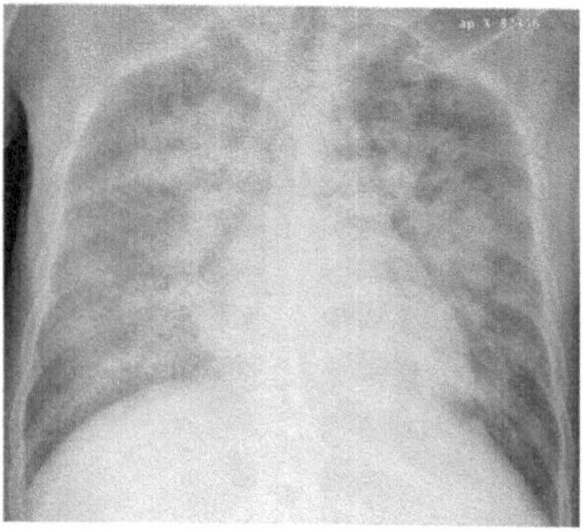

Figure 2.23: Chest radiograph showing inhomogeneous air space opacities in bilateral lungs in a case of pulmonary edema

SOLITARY PULMONARY NODULE (SPN)

Findings on Chest X-Ray:

SPN is defined as a nodule which is relatively well-defined, round or oval in shape, surrounded at least partially by lung parenchyma, less than 3 cm in diameter and is not associated with lymphadenopathy, atelectasis or pneumonia.

Causes:

Infective

Congenital lesions (bronchogenic cyst, CCAM, sequestration, intrapulmonary lymph node).

Benign Neoplasms (hamartoma, mesenchymal tumor).

Malignancy

Inflammatory (rheumatoid nodules, sarcoidosis, Wegener's granulomatosis).

Airway and Inhalational diseases (mucoid impaction, bronchial atresia, cystic fibrosis).

Vascular lesions (hematoma, infarction, pulmonary artery aneurysm, septic embolism).

Miscellaneous (amyloidosis, fluid filled bulla, round atelectasis).

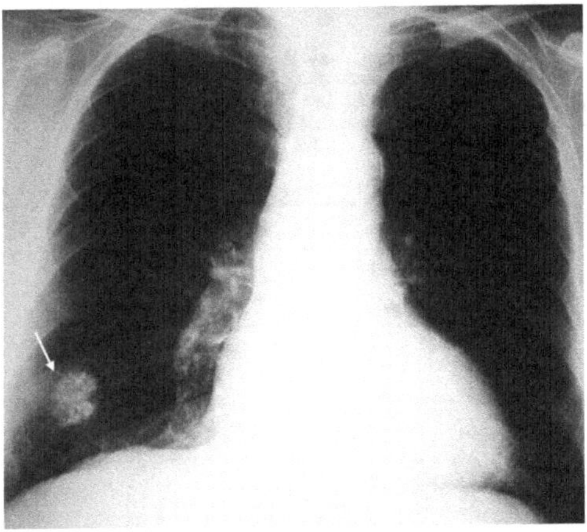

Figure 2.24: Chest radiograph showing solitary pulmonary nodule (arrow) in right lower zone

MEDIASTINUM

Boundaries of Mediastinum on Lateral Chest X-Ray According to Felson:

Anterior: Part of mediastinum lying between line drawn along anterior border of trachea to posterior border of the heart (First line).

Middle: Part of mediastinum lying between First line and line joining a point 1 cm behind the anterior margins of dorsal vertebrae (Second line).

Posterior: Part of mediastinum behind the Second line.

Common mediastinal masses		
Anterior	**Middle**	**Posterior**
Teratoma-germ cell tumors	Lymph nodes	Neurogenic tumors
Thymic tumor	Bronchogenic cyst	Duplication cysts
Lymphoma	Aneurysm of aortic arch	Extramedullary haematopoiesis
Retrosternal thyroid		Rhabdomyosarcoma
Lymhangioma		Vascular malformations
Pericardial cysts		Lymph nodes
Aneurysm of ascending aorta		Abscess
		Aneurysm of descending aorta

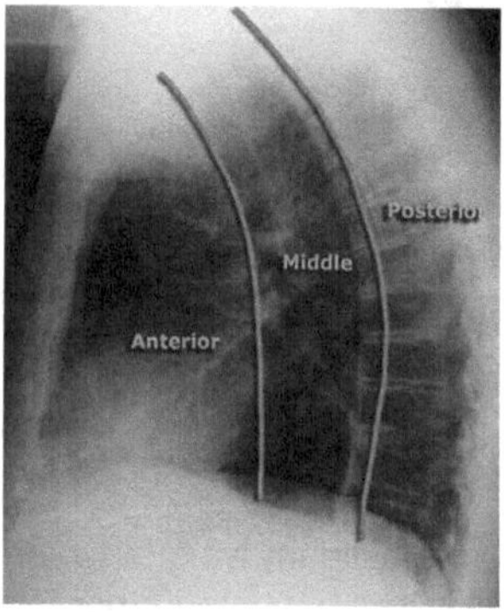

Figure 2.25: Lateral chest radiograph showing divisions of mediastinum

Differentiating Pulmonary, Mediastinal, Pleural and Extra-pleural Lesions

Pulmonary	Mediastinum	Pleural	Extrapleural
May contain air bronchogram	Air broncho-gram absent	Air broncho-gram absent	Air broncho-gram absent
Acute angle with the lung if abutting the mediastinum	Obtuse margins with lung	Obtuse angle; lesion located peripherally	Obtuse angle
Mediastinal lines not displaced	Mediastinal lines displaced	Mediastinal lines not displaced	Mediastinal lines not displaced
Usually no bony destruction	Bony destruc-tion may be seen	Rib erosion unusual	Rib erosion always
One side of hemithorax	May extend to both sides of hemithorax	One side of hemithorax	One side of hemithorax
Engulfs pulmo-nary vasculature	Displaces pulmonary vasculature	Displaces pulmonary vasculature	Displaces pulmonary vasculature
Lesion centred in lung	Centred in the mediastinum	Centred along chest wall	Lesion centred along chest wall
Ill-defined non-tapering margins	Tapered well-defined lateral margins and medial margins merging with the mediastinum	Tapered well-defined medial margins	Tapered well-defined medial margins

PULMONARY TUBERCULOSIS

Primary Tuberculosis

- Patchy areas or consolidation or even lobar consolidation (Radiographic evidence of parenchymal infection is seen in 70% of children and 90% of adults).

- Cavitation is uncommon in primary TB, seen only in 10-30% of cases. In most cases the infection becomes localised and a caseating granuloma forms (tuberculoma) which usually eventually calcifies, and is then known as a Ghon lesion.

The more striking finding, especially in children, is that of ipsilateral hilar and contiguous mediastinal (paratracheal) lymphadenopathy, usually right sided. This pattern is seen in over 90% of cases of childhood primary TB, but only 10-30% of adults. These nodes typically have low density centres with rim enhancement on CT. Occasionally these nodes may be large enough to compress adjacent airways resulting in distal atelectasis.

Pleural effusions are more frequent in adults, seen in 30-40% of cases, whereas they are only present in 5-10% of paediatric cases. As the host mounts an appropriate immune response both the pulmonary and nodal disease resolves. Calcification of nodes is seen in 35% of cases. When a calcified node and a Ghon lesion are present, the combination is known as a Ranke complex.

Post-Primary Pulmonary Tuberculosis

Post-primary TB, also known as reactivation TB or secondary TB occurs years later, frequently in the setting of a decreased immune status. In the majority of cases, post-primary TB within the lungs develops in either:

1. Posterior segments of the upper lobes.
2. Superior segments of the lower lobes.

Typical appearance of post primary TB is that of patchy consolidation or poorly defined linear and nodular opacities. Post-primary infections are far more likely to cavitate than primary infections, and are seen in 20-45% of cases. In the vast majority of cases they develop in the posterior segments of the upper lobes. The development of an air-fluid level implies communication with the airway, and thus the possibility of contagion. Endobronchial spread along nearby airways is a relatively common finding, resulting in relatively well-defined 2-4 mm nodules or branching lesions tree-in-bud appearance on CT. Hilar nodal enlargement is seen in only approximately a third of cases. Lobar consolidation, tuberculoma formation and miliary TB are also recognised patterns of post-primary TB but are less common.

Miliary Tuberculosis

Miliary tuberculosis is uncommon but carries a poor prognosis. It represents haematogeneous dissemination of an uncontrolled tuberculous infection. It is seen both in primary and post-primary tuberculosis. Miliary deposits appear as 1-3 mm diameter nodules, which are uniform in size and uniformly distributed. If treatment is successful no residual abnormality remains.

Tracheal and Bronchial Involvement

Isolated tracheal infection by tuberculosis is rare, but reported and typically results in irregular circumferential mural thickening. It is usually the result of contiguous inflammation from adjacent nodal involvement.

Broncholith

A broncholith is a relatively uncommon presentation which is due to erosion of a calcified lymph node into a bronchus, resulting in calcified material entering the lumen. Rarely this material can be coughed-up (known as lithoptysis).

Complications of Pulmonary Tuberculosis

Aspergilloma.

Empyema.

Fibrothorax.

Bronchopleural fistula.

Arterial pseudoaneurysm – bronchial artery, pulmonary artery (Rasmussen aneurysm).

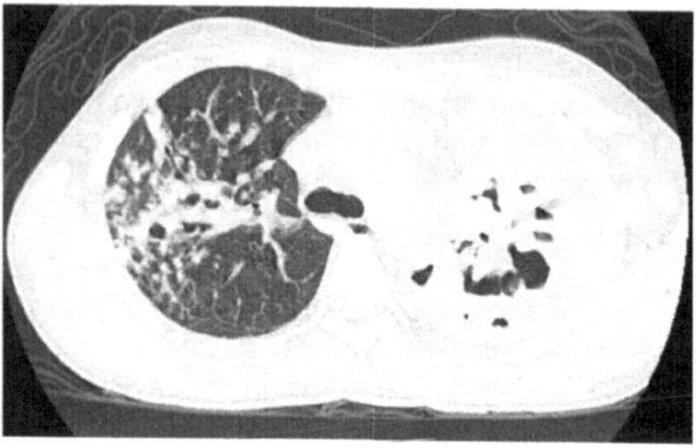

Figure 2.26: Axial CT chest showing consolidation with breakdown in bilateral upper lobes with nodules showing tree-in-bud appearance in right upper lobe in a case of pulmonary tuberculosis

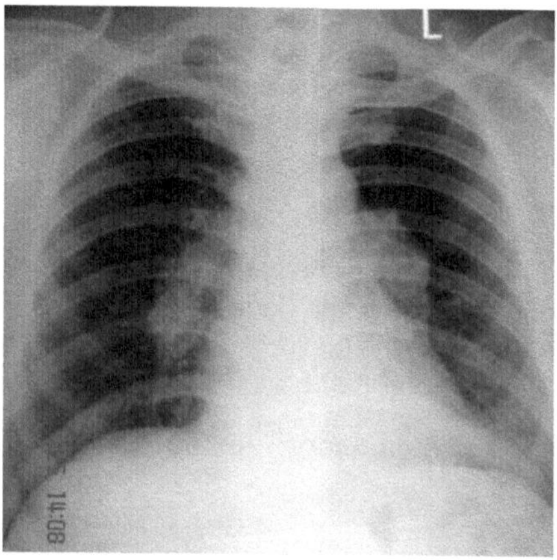

Figure 2.27: Chest radiograph showing bilateral hilar masses with lobulated lateral margins suggestive of hilar lymphadenopathy (DD: Tuberculosis, sarcoidosis, lymphoma)

PLEUROPULMONARY BLASTOMA

Pleuropulmonary blastoma (PPB) is a rare malignant embryonal mesenchymal neoplasm of the lung and pleura-occurring almost exclusively in children.

Type I: Purely cystic.

Type II: Solid-cystic.

Type III: Purely solid.

Imaging:

X-Ray: Unilateral white out lung with mediastinal shift to opposite side. Usually there is no adjacent rib erosions or calcification.

CT

Large mass in the thorax with solid-cystic heterogeneous enhancement with contralateral mediastinal shift, and lack of chest wall invasion, may be associated with pleural effusion rarely.

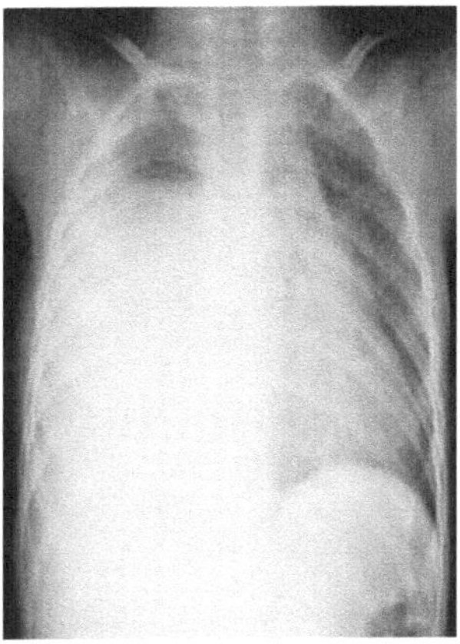

Figure 2.28: Chest radiograph showing homogeneous opacity in right hemithorax causing mediastinal shift to the left side

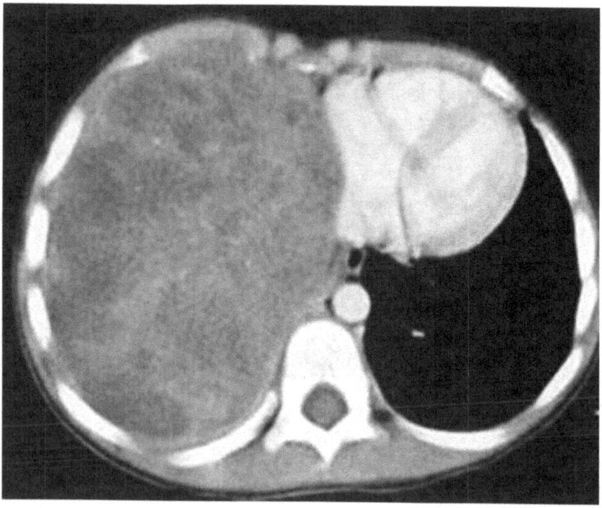

Figure 2.29: Axial contrast-enhanced CT scan image showing heterogenously enhancing mass lesion in right lungs causing mediastinal shift to left with no bony erosion in a case of pleuropulmonary blastoma

TUMORS METASTASIZING TO LUNGS IN CHILDREN

1. Wilm's tumor.
2. Osteosarcoma.
3. Ewing's sarcoma.
4. Rhabdomyosarcoma.
5. Lymphoma.
6. Leukaemia.
7. Neuroblastoma.
8. Germ cell tumors.

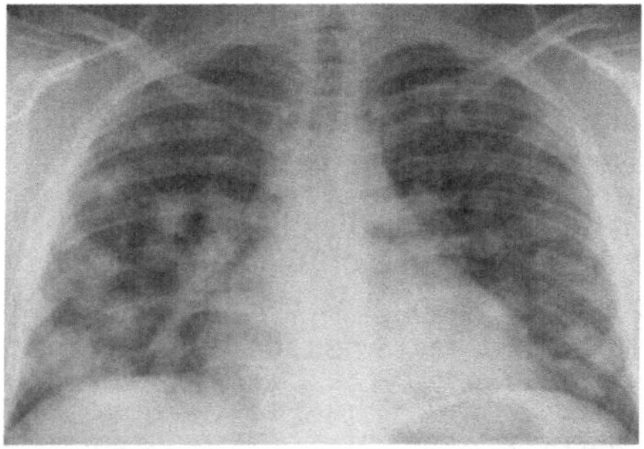

Figure 2.30: Chest radiograph showing multiple nodules of variable sizes in bilateral lungs suggestive of metastases from osteosarcoma of femur

LUNG HYDATID

Imaging:

Multiple or solitary cystic lesion (most common), diameter of 1-20 cm, unilateral or bilateral, predominantly found in the lower lobes.

Uncomplicated cysts are characterized by round or oval masses with well-defined borders, enhancement after contrast injection, and hypodense content relative to the capsule.

Complicated cysts may show meniscus sign or air crescent sign, cumbo sign or onion peel sign, water-lily sign, consolidation adjacent to the cyst (ruptured cyst).

Signs:

Cumbo sign: Air is seen between the pericyst and the laminated membrane of the cyst.

Serpent sign: Internal rupture of the cyst with collapse of membranes of parasite into the cyst.

Spin sign: Detached membranes with small pleural reaction seen in hydatid cyst of lung.

Empty cyst sign: May be seen after complete evacuation of parasitic membranes.

Crescent sign: A crescent-shaped rim of air at the lower end of the cyst (inverse crescent sign).

Waterlily sign: Floating membranes within the pericyst that mimic the appearance of a water lily. It may be seen on ultrasound and CT-scan. It is classically described on plain films (mainly chest X-ray) when the collapsed membranes are calcified.

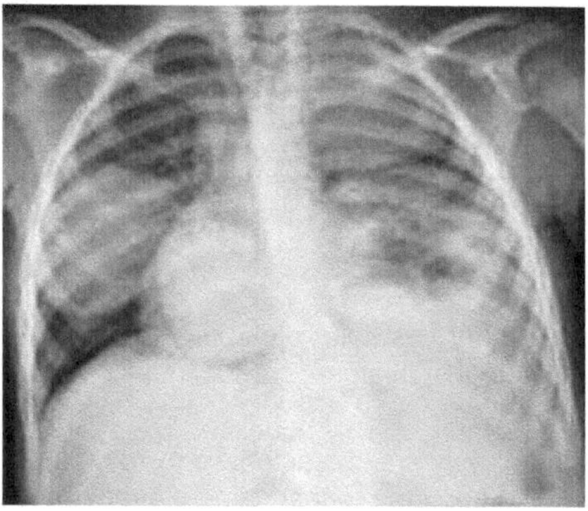

Figure 2.31: Chest radiograph showing multiple well-defined lesions in bilateral lungs in a case of hydatid disease of lungs

3

Chapter

Cardiac X-Rays Interpretation

1. Situs:

The term situs refers to the position of the heart and viscera relative to midline.

Normally, the liver, inferior vena cava lies on the right side and gastric fundus and spleen lies on the left side. Systemic venous atrium lies on the right and opposite the gastric fundus. This relationship is referred to as "viscero-atrial situs".

Situs solitus refers to normal configuration of abdominal and thoracic organs. It denotes that the liver, right atrium, inferior vena cava and right bronchus is on right side and gastric fundus, cardiac apex, aorta, spleen, left sided bronchus on the left side.

Situs inversus *is mirror image of normal.*

Situs inversus is divided into situs inversus with dextrocardia and situs inversus with levocardia. Situs inversus with dextrocardia is more common and is characterized by mirror image location of the heart and viscera relative to situs solitus, with the cardiac apex, spleen, stomach, and aorta located on the right and the liver and inferior vena cava located on the left. Congenital heart disease occurs in 3%–5% of cases. In contrast, situs inversus with levocardia is an extremely rare variant that is characterized by mirror-image location of the viscera relative to situs solitus and a left-sided cardiac apex. Nearly all affected individuals have congenital heart disease.

Situs inversus totalis is total transposition of abdominal and thoracic viscera (mirror image of internal organs normal positioning).

***Situs ambiguous**, also known as heterotaxia syndromes is an intermediate configuration with duplication (isomerism).* The two major subcategories of situs ambiguous are situs ambiguous with polysplenia and situs ambiguous with asplenia. Situs ambiguous with polysplenia (left isomerism or bilateral left-sidedness) is characterized in general by midline or ambiguous location of the majority of the abdominal organs and multiple spleens. Situs ambiguous with asplenia (right isomerism or bilateral right-sidedness) is characterized by ambiguous location of the abdominal organs and absence of the spleen. Patients of situs ambiguous with asplenia have a 99%–100% prevalence of congenital heart disease that is much more severe than that seen with polysplenia and the other situs anomalies.

2. Cardiac Contour

AP view: The right border of the cardiac silhouette is formed by the following structures from top to bottom: superior vena cava, ascending aorta, right atrial appendage, right atrium and inferior vena cava. The left border of the cardiac silhouette is formed from top to bottom by the aortic arch (aortic knob), pulmonary trunk, left atrial appendage, and the left ventricle. The right ventricle does not contribute to either heart border.

Lateral view: The ascending aorta, right atrial appendage and right ventricle form the anterior border, while the left atrium and left ventricle forms the posterior border.

3. Cardiac Size

The cardiac silhouette occupies 50–55% of the chest width. Cardiomegaly is present when the cardiothoracic ratio is more than 55% in infants and more than 60% in neonates.

4. Chamber Enlargement

Right Atrium	Left Atrium	Right Ventricle	Left Ventricle
Right heart border more convex	Enlarges posteriorly and to the right displacing the esophagus posteriorly	Enlarges to the left and anteriorly	Enlarges to the left and posteriorly
Maximum convexity of right cardiac border more than 3 cm beyond the right lateral vertebral border	Lifting of the left main bronchus	Elevation of cardiac apex	Cardiac apex shifts downwards and to the left
Distance between top of aortic arch and junction of the SVC with right atrium is less than distance between the latter and right cardiophrenic angle	Widening of carinal angle (Normal : 51-71 degrees) Double density shadow on frontal radiograph	Pulmonary conus becomes prominent while aortic knuckle is less prominent On lateral radiograph there is obliteration of upper retrosternal space	

5. Pulmonary Vasculature

In normal individuals, the pulmonary arteries in outer one-third of lungs are usually not seen. In children, the ratio of right descending pulmonary artery (RDPA) to trachea is <1. The lower lobe vessels are 2-3 times larger than upper lobe vessels. In an erect chest radiograph, vessels in the first intercostal space are <3 mm in diameter and those just above the diaphragm are up to 6 mm in diameter.

Pulmonary Plethora	**Pulmonary Oligemia**
Seen in left to right shunts	Seen in right to left shunts
End on vessels are more than twice the diameter of accompanying bronchus	Concave or absent pulmonary artery at hila
Vessels seen below the 10th posterior rib	Over-penetrated film
Vessels seen behind and below the diaphragm	< 4 vessels in outer-third of lungs
RDPA diameter more than trachea	Small hila
>6 vessels in outer-third of lungs	Enlarged bronchial and systemic arteries
RDPA > 16 mm in diameter	
Prominent hilar vessels	
Generalized mottling of lungs	

Pulmonary Arterial Hypertension	**Pulmonary Venous Hypertension**
Centrally enlarged pulmonary arteries and pruning of pulmonary arteries in the periphery	Stage 1: Cephalization of blood flow (13-19 mm Hg)
Pruning is defined as > 50% reduction in vessel diameter	Stage 2: Interstitial edema (20-24 mm Hg)
	Stage 3: Alveolar edema (25 mm Hg and above)

6. Aorta

Aortic knuckle right or left sided, aorta normal, small or enlarged.

<table>
<tr><th>Pulmonary Plethora</th><th>Pulmonary Oligemia</th></tr>
<tr><td>Pulmonary plethora with large aorta: PDA, ruptured aneurysm of sinus of valsalva, Aortopulmonary window, coronary arteriovenous fistula</td><td>Pulmonary oligemia with large aorta: Tetralogy of Fallot (TOF), pulmonary atresia with VSD, tricuspid atresia, double outlet right ventricles with pulmonary stenosis, TGA with VSD and PS.</td></tr>
<tr><td>Normal aorta with pulmonary plethora: ASD, VSD and partial anomalous pulmonary venous drainage</td><td rowspan="3">Normal aorta with pulmonary oligemia: Ebstein's anomaly, valvular PS</td></tr>
<tr><td>Small aorta with pulmonary plethora: TGA</td></tr>
<tr><td>Large pedicle with pulmonary plethora: Truncus arteriosus, TAPVC and tricuspid atresia without PS</td></tr>
</table>

Clinical and Radiological Classification of Congenital Heart Diseases

Acyanotic CHD	
Increased Pulmonary Vasculature	***Normal Pulmonary Vasculature***
VSD	Coarctation of aorta
PDA	Congenital aortic stenosis
ASD	Congenital pulmonary stenosis
PAPVC	
AV canal defect	
Cyanotic CHD	
Increased Pulmonary Vasculature	***Decreased Pulmonary Vasculature***
TGA	TOF
TAPVC (Supradiaphragmatic type)	Ebstein's anomaly
Truncus arteriosus	Tricuspid atresia

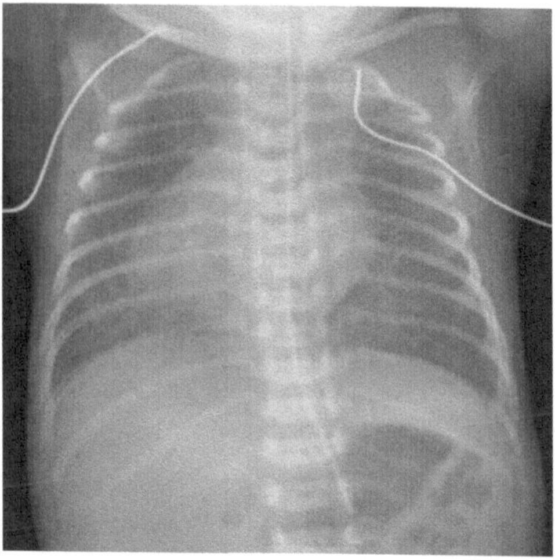

Figure 3.1: Chest radiograph showing situs solitus with dextrocardia

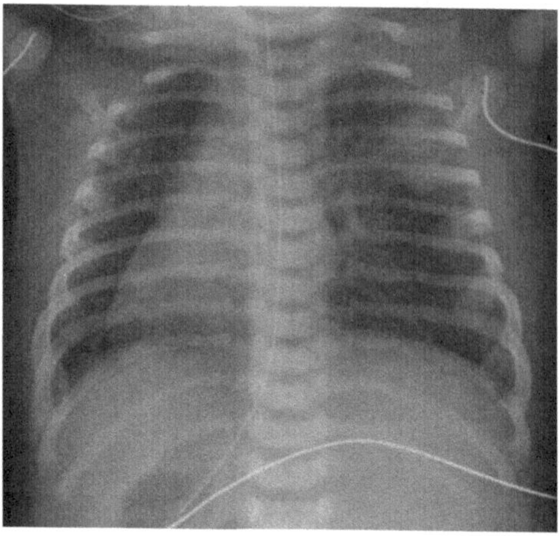

Figure 3.2: Chest radiograph showing situs inversus with dextrocardia

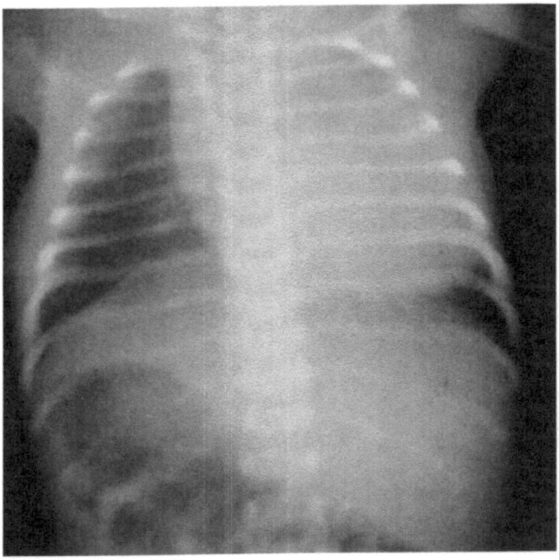

Figure 3.3: Chest radiograph showing situs inversus with levocardia

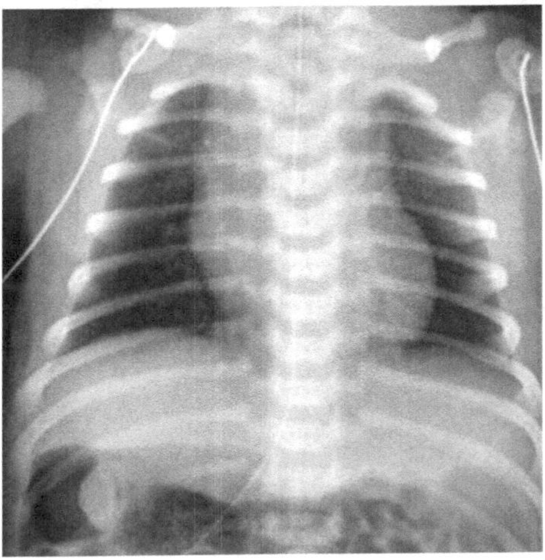

Figure 3.4: Chest radiograph showing situs ambiguous with midline liver

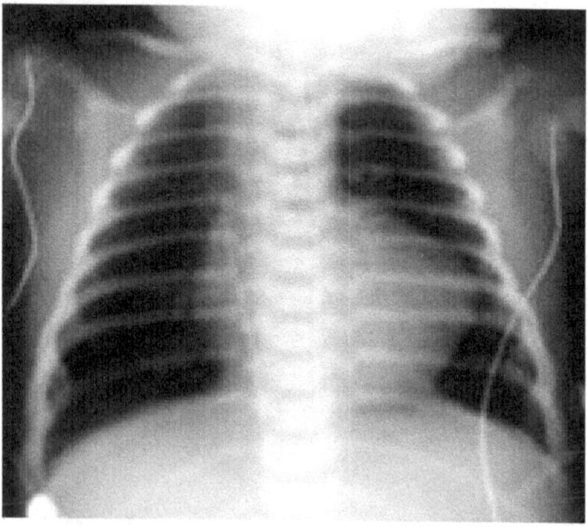

Figure 3.5: Chest radiograph showing pulmonary oligemia

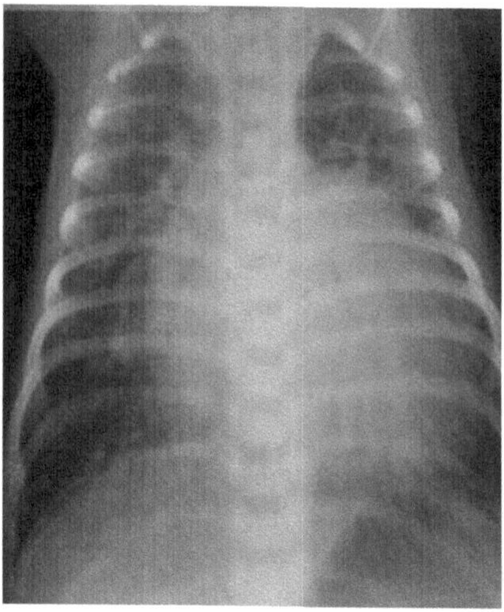

Figure 3.6: Chest radiograph showing pulmonary plethora and cardiomegaly

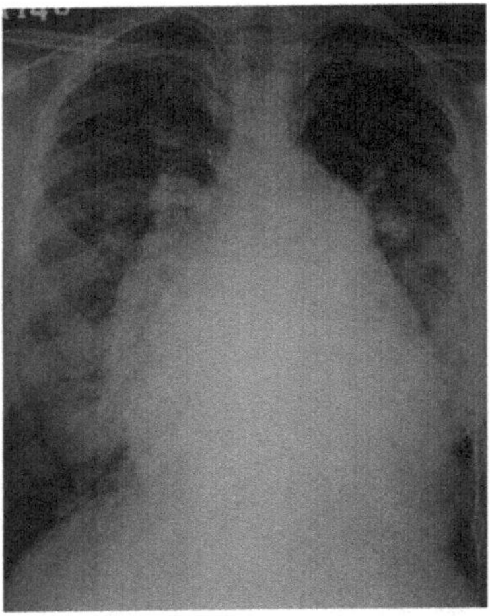

Figure 3.7: Chest radiograph of a case of ventricular septal defect showing pulmonary plethora and mild cardiomegaly in a case of VSD

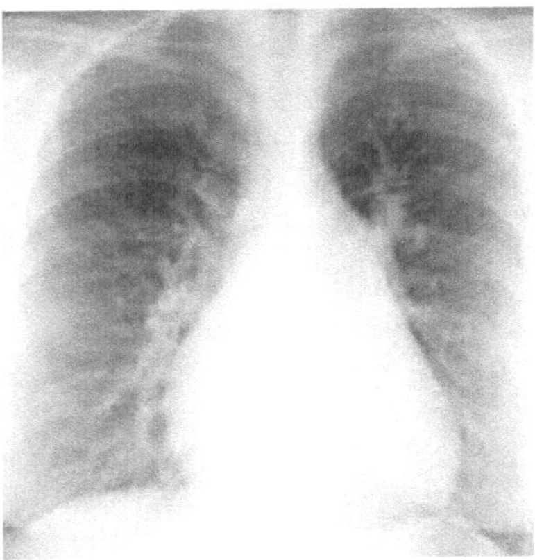

Figure 3.8: Chest radiograph of a case of atrial septal defect showing normal sized aorta, mild pulmonary plethora and fullness of pulmonary bay

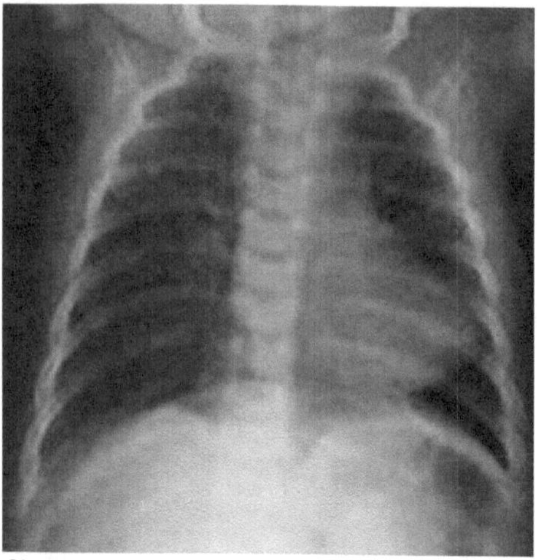

Figure 3.9: Chest radiograph showing boot shaped heart and pulmonary oligemia in a case of Tetralogy of Fallot

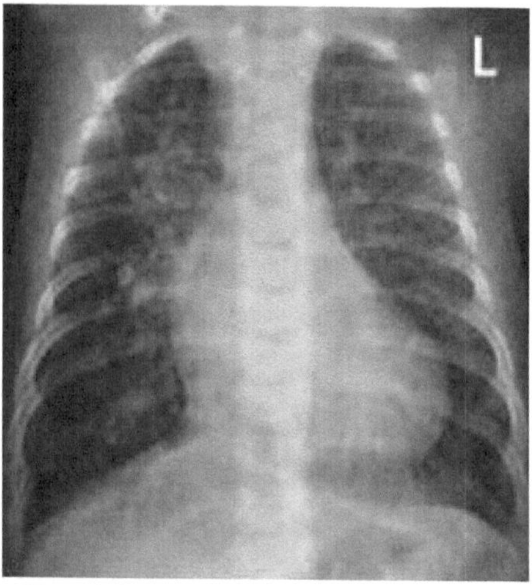

Figure 3.10: Chest radiograph showing pulmonary plethora, small aorta and 'egg on string' appearance in a case of TGA

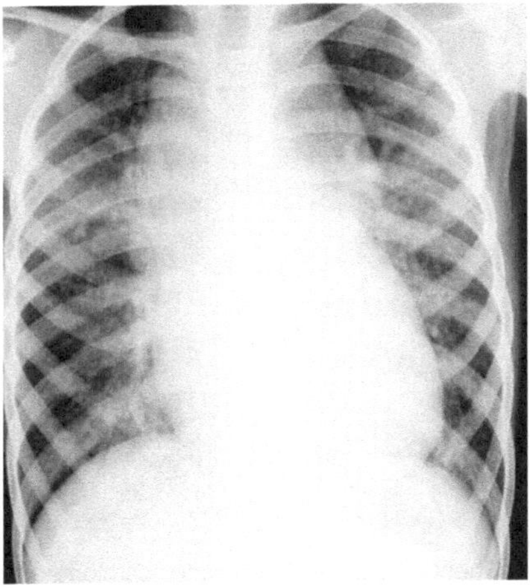

Figure 3.11: Chest radiograph showing 'snowman sign' in a case of TAPVC

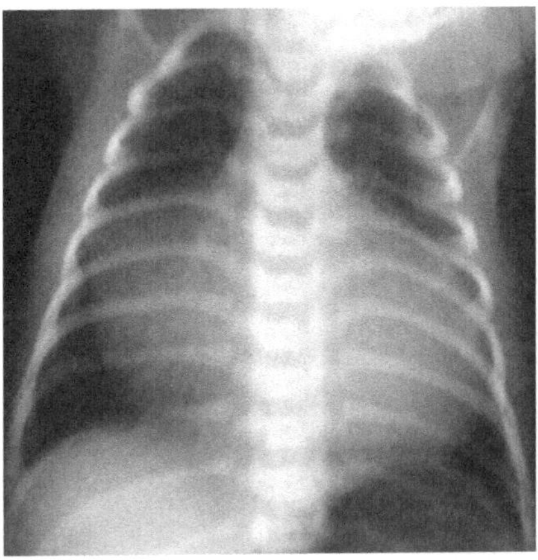

Figure 3.12: Chest radiograph showing pulmonary oligemia, enlarged right atrium and a box-shape heart in a case of Ebstein's anomaly

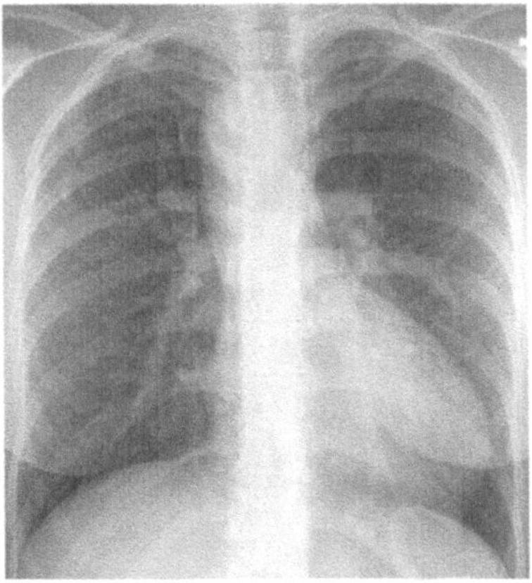

Figure 3.13: Chest radiograph showing cardiomegaly, pulmonary plethora and a large pedicle in a case of truncus arteriosus

4

Chapter

Gastrointestinal Tract

ESOPHAGEAL ATRESIA AND TRACHEOESOPHAGEAL FISTULA (TEF)

Classification

Type A–Esophageal atresia without fistula (7.8%)

Type B–Esophageal atresia with proximal fistula (0.8%)

Type C–Esophageal atresia with distal fistula (85.8%)

Type D–Esophageal atresia with fistula in both proximal and distal ends (1.4%)

Type E–H-type fistula without atresia (4.2%).

Imaging Findings

Frontal radiograph showing dilated proximal esophageal pouch with round distal margin and coiled nasogastric tube within is diagnostic of esophageal atresia. The presence of air in the stomach and small bowel indicates esophageal atresia with a distal tracheoesophageal fistula. Absence of air in stomach excludes presence of distal fistula. In addition, if air is only confined to the stomach, the possibility of coexisting duodenal atresia should also be considered.

When type E (H-shaped tracheoesophageal fistula without atresia) is suspected, radiologic investigation is directed toward demonstration of the fistula, which typically courses forward and upward from the esophagus. Non-ionic water-soluble contrast material is preferable in these patients.

Most of the H-type fistula occurs at the level of thoracic inlet, between C7 and D2 vertebral bodies. The fistulous connection is angulated superiorly from the esophagus to the trachea.

The best technique of demonstrating the fistula is by careful injection of contrast via a feeding tube, first placed at gastro-esophageal junction and then gradually withdrawing the tube with simultaneous injection of contrast under fluoroscopic guidance.

The side of aortic arch should also be identified as the surgical approach is from the side opposite the aortic arch.

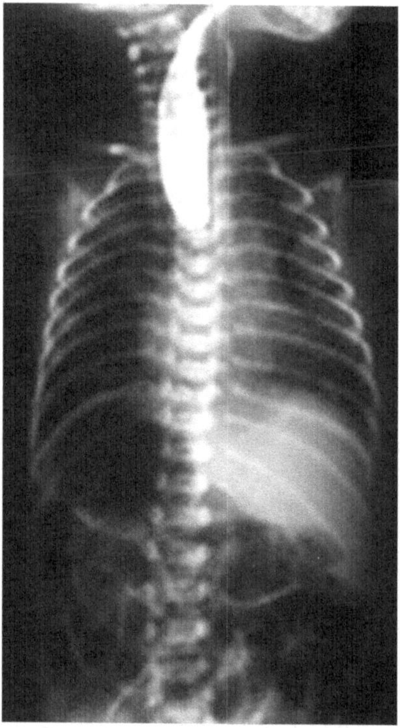

Figure 4.1: Esophagram study showing esophageal atresia with distal fistula. Also note is made of situs inversus with dextrocardia

ACHALASIA CARDIA

Imaging Findings

Chest X-ray

Convex opacity on the right side behind right cardiac border, air-fluid level due to stasis in thoracic esophagus filled with retained secretions and food, small/absent gastric air bubble.

Barium Swallow

Failure of normal peristalsis to clear the esophagus of barium when the patient is in the recumbent position, uncoordinated, non-propulsive, tertiary contractions, esophageal body dilatation, which is typically maximal in the distal esophagus, incomplete relaxation of lower esophageal sphincter.

Bird beak sign–Beak like narrowing at lower esophageal sphincter.

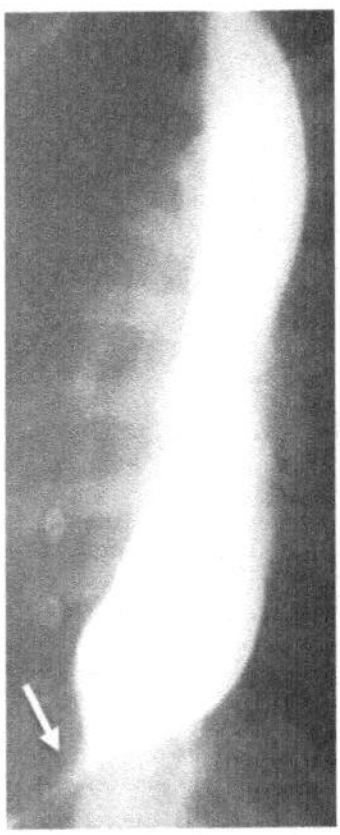

Figure 4.2: Contrast esophagram study showing dilated esophagus and bird-beak appearance of lower esophageal sphincter

HYPERTROPHIC PYLORIC STENOSIS (HPS)

Imaging Findings

Ultrasonography

Performed with a high frequency linear transducer. The stomach should not be empty prior to the examination. If there is inadequate distension, the infant may be given a glucose solution or water orally by a feeding tube.

The pyloric muscle thickness (diameter of a single muscular wall on a transverse image) more than **3 mm** (most accurate), transverse serosa-to-serosa diameter more than 15 mm and the length (longitudinal measurement) more than **15 mm** is diagnostic for HPS.

Barium Study

Barium study reveals delayed gastric emptying.

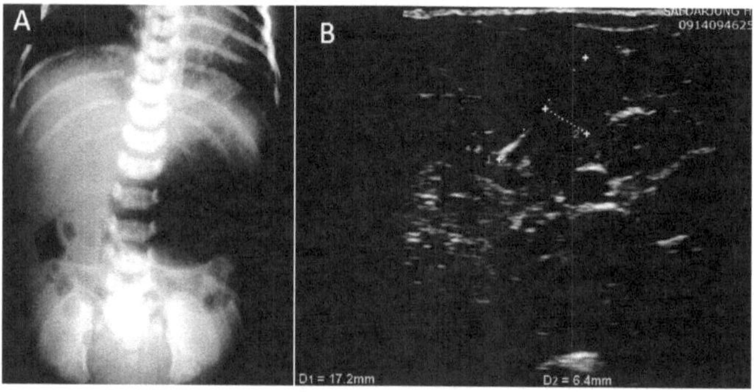

Figure 4.3: (A) Plain X-ray abdomen showing distended stomach with paucity of gases in distal bowel loops (B) Ultrasound image of a case of hypertrophic pyloric stenosis showing thickened pyloric muscle

String sign – Pyloric canal narrowed and elongated.

Double-tract sign – Barium caught in the folds and appearing as parallel lines.

Shoulder sign – Hypertophied pylorus indents the contrast-filled gastric antrum.

Mushroom sign – Hypertrophied pylorus indenting the base of the duodenal bulb.

Beak sign – Narrowing of barium column as it enters the pyloric canal.

ANOMALIES OF ROTATION AND FIXATION

1. *Nonrotation* – Asymptomatic condition in which small bowel lies on the right side and the colon on left side.
2. *Malrotation* – Incomplete rotation, associated with midgut volvulus and Ladd's bands.
3. *Reversed intestinal rotation* – Rare anomaly in which hepatic flexure and distal transverse colon lies posterior to the second part of duodenum and SMA. Caecum is malrotated and medially placed, small bowel is predominantly on the right side.

Imaging Findings

Plain radiographs may show features of duodenal obstruction due to obstructing Ladd's bands with little distal bowel gas. Bowel wall thickening and pneumatosis may be seen when there is ischaemia due to volvulus.

Barium Examination

The normal position of the duodenojejunal (DJ) junction is to the left of the left-sided pedicles of the vertebral body at the level of the duodenal bulb on frontal views and posterior (retroperitoneal) on lateral views.

In children with acute duodenal obstruction, the upper GI study may depict a Z-shaped configuration of the duodenum in the presence of obstructing peritoneal bands or a corkscrew-shaped duodenum in the presence of volvulus. In children who have bowel malrotation without volvulus, the upper GI study shows an abnormal position of the DJ junction.

Ultrasonography and CT

Dilated duodenum, fluid and edematous bowel loops may be seen. Abnormal SMA, SMV relationship may be seen. SMV to the left of SMA is highly suggestive of volvulus. When SMV is anterior to the SMA, it is suggestive of malrotation with possible volvulus. Color Doppler ultrasound shows 'whirlpool sign' due to clockwise spiralling of the SMV around the SMA.

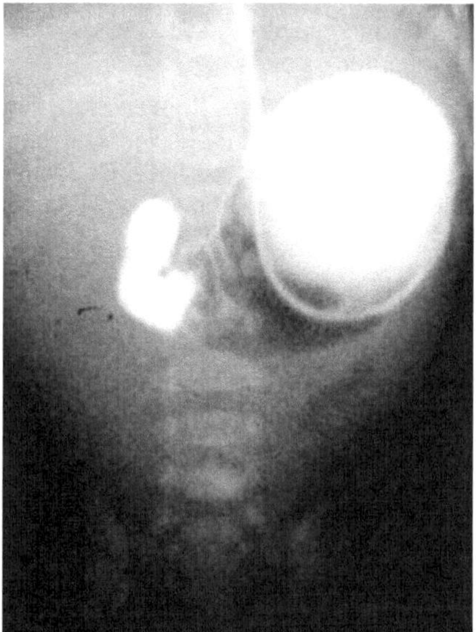

Figure 4.4: Barium examination showing DJ flexure on the right side with cork-screw appearance of duodenum in a case of malrotation with volvulus

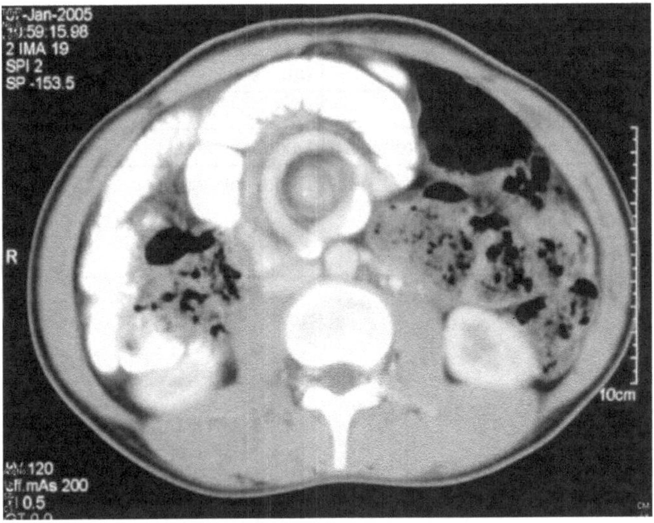

Figure 4.5: Axial contrast CT scan image showing whirlpool sign in a case of malrotation with volvulus

DUODENAL ATRESIA AND STENOSIS

Imaging Findings

Plain abdominal radiograph is diagnostic. The typical appearance of "double-bubble sign" is characteristic of duodenal atresia. This represents air in the stomach and duodenal bulb and absence of air in the distal bowel. In duodenal stenosis, air is also present in the distal bowel.

"Single bubble sign" is characteristic of gastric atresia.

Causes of Duodenal Obstruction in Newborn:

Extrinsic	Intrinsic
Ladd's bands	Duodenal web
Midgut volvulus with malrotation	Duodenal atresia
Annular pancreas	Duodenal stenosis
Duplication anomalies	
Preduodenal portal vein	

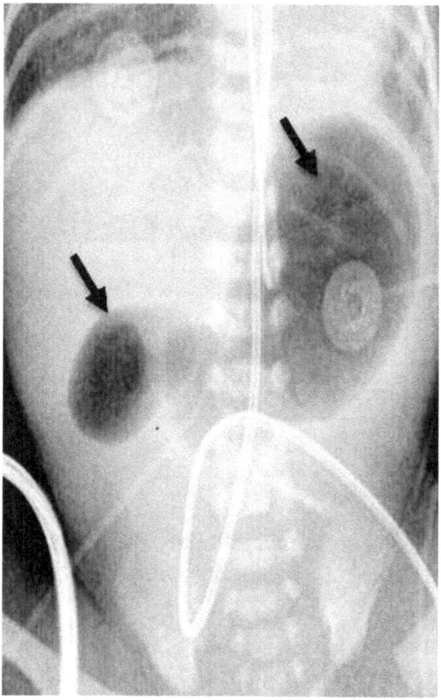

Figure 4.6: Radiograph of the abdomen in a newborn showing double-bubble sign in a case of duodenal atresia

JEJUNAL ATRESIA

Imaging Findings

Plain abdominal radiograph demonstrates findings of small-bowel obstruction. "Triple bubble sign" is characteristic of proximal jejunal atresia. In distal jejunal atresia, there is more uniform dilatation of small bowel with air-fluid levels.

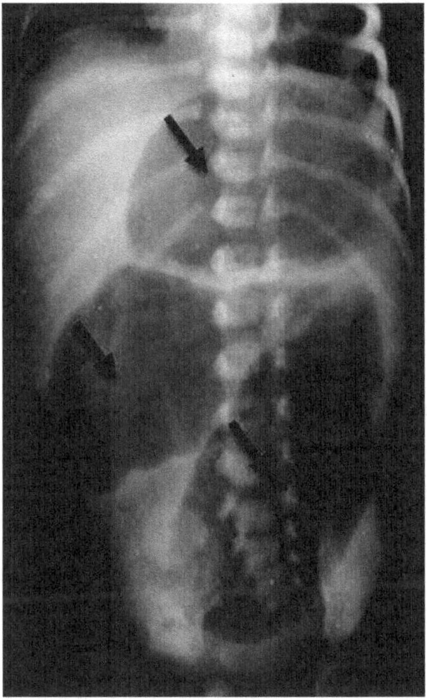

Figure 4.7: Radiograph of the abdomen in a newborn showing triple-bubble sign in a case of jejunal atresia

INTUSSUSCEPTION

Sites: Ileocolic–most common (75-95%), followed by ileocolic, ileoileal and colocolic.

Imaging Findings

Plain radiographs: The role of plain radiography in intussusception is to exclude intussusception and diagnose other pathologic processes that are responsible for the patient's symptoms, confirm the diagnosis of intussusception and if intussusception is present, the role of plain radiography is to identify intestinal obstruction or perforation.

Findings on abdominal radiograph are soft-tissue mass (most often seen in the right upper quadrant effacing the adjacent hepatic contour), reduced air in the small intestine or a gasless abdomen, absence of caecal gas and obstruction of the small intestine. Most specific findings are the target sign and meniscus sign.

Target sign–Soft-tissue mass containing concentric circular area of lucency due to the mesenteric fat of the intussusceptum.

Meniscus sign–Crescent of gas within the colonic lumen that outlines the apex of the intussusceptum.

Identification of a cecum filled with gas or feces in the normal location excludes intussusception.

Ultrasonography

Mass with atypical target or a concentric ring appearance in transverse section and *sandwich/pseudokidney* appearance in sagittal plane. Characteristic appearance of eccentric, echogenic mesenteric fat on transverse section with pulled mesenteric vessels and lymph nodes. On color Doppler, absence of color flow indicates ischemia and necrosis.

Barium Enema

Barium enema examination is the gold standard investigation for intussusception.

Meniscus sign–Analogous to the meniscus sign at plain radiography and is produced by the rounded apex of the intussusceptum protruding into the column of contrast material.

Coiled spring sign–Edematous mucosal folds of the returning limb of the intussusceptum is outlined by contrast material in the lumen of the colon.

CT: Bowel-within-bowel configuration.

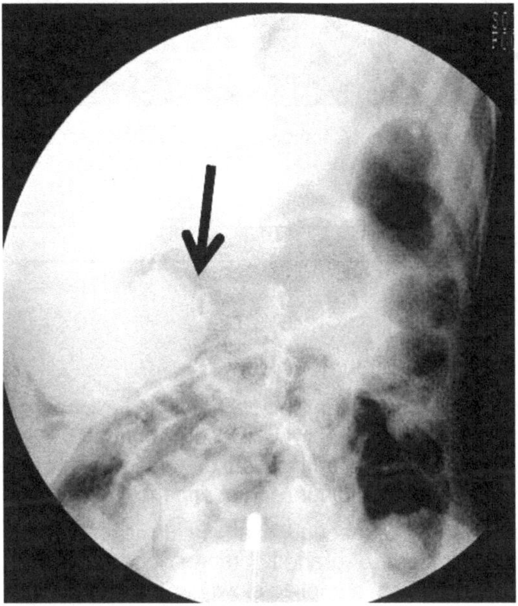

Figure 4.8: Plain abdomen X-ray showing 'meniscus sign' due to intussusceptum protruding into the large bowel

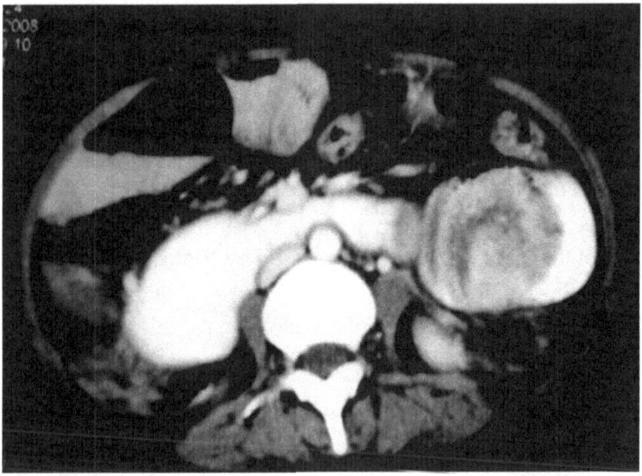

Figure 4.9: Axial contrast CT showing bowel-within-bowel configuration in a case of intussusception

APPENDICITIS

Imaging Findings

Plain Abdominal Radiograph

Mass effect on the caecum, air-fluid level in terminal ileum and caecum, thickened caecum wall, loss of obturator internus fat plane, Appendicolith. Identification of Appendicolith in a child with acute abdomen is diagnostic of appendicitis.

Ultrasonography: Ultrasound examination is performed using a specific technique of graded compression. In this technique, graded compression is applied slowly and gently, similar to the classic palpation of the abdomen which displaces the fat and bowel. This eliminates the disturbing influence of bowel gas and reduces the distance from the transducer to the appendix.

Inflamed, tubular, non-compressible, aperistaltic, blind ending structure with diameter > 6 mm, periappendiceal fluid, Appendicolith and appendiceal abscess.

CT:

Dilated appendix with distended lumen (> 6 mm diameter).

Caecal bar sign – Inflammatory soft tissue at the base of the appendix that separates the appendix from the contrast-filled cecum.

Arrowhead sign – Enteric contrast material in the caecal lumen points to the abnormal appendix and assuming a triangular configuration, mimicking an arrowhead.

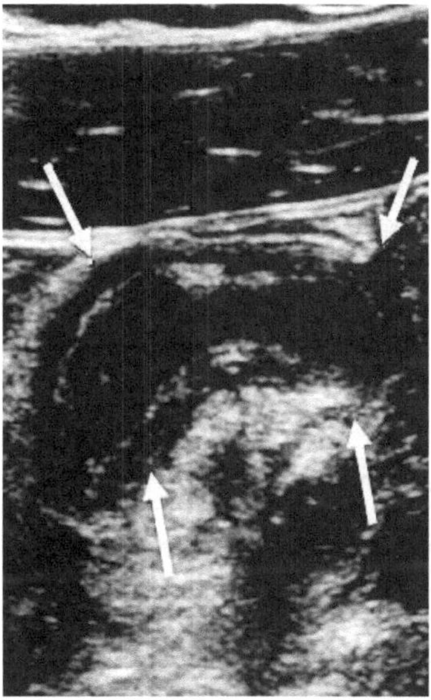

Figure 4.10: Ultrasound showing tubular, aperistaltic blind ending structure in a case of acute appendicitis with surrounding inflammatory changes in mesenteric fat and mild periappendiceal fluid

ABDOMINAL TUBERCULOSIS

Imaging Findings

Plain radiograph: Presence of multiple air-fluid levels and dilated bowel loops which suggests obstruction, enteroliths calcified lymph nodes. Radiograph of chest may show evidence of active or healed pulmonary tuberculosis in some patients.

Barium Meal Follow Through (BMFT)

Multiple strictures, mucosal irregularity and rapid emptying (ulcerative), flocculation and fragmentation of barium (malabsorption), dilated loops and strictures, displaced loops (due to enlarged lymph nodes), adherent fixed loops (adhesive peritoneal disease).

Fleischner sign–Thickening of the ileocaecal valve lips and/or wide gaping of the valve with narrowing of the terminal ileum.

Goose neck deformity–Retracted, conical caecum resulting in loss of normal ileocaecal angle resulting in suspension of dilated terminal ileum.

Stierlin's sign–Narrowing of terminal ileum due to irritability with rapid emptying through a gaping ileocaecal valve with short and rigid caecum (represents acute on chronic inflammation).

String sign–Narrow stream of barium indication stenosis.

Ultrasound and CT

Ileocaecal thickening, nodular or symmetrical thickening of the peritoneum and mesentery, abnormal peritoneal or mesenteric enhancement, ascites (with internal echoes and septations on ultrasound) and enlarged lymph nodes of low attenuation due to necrosis.

Types:

Wet type	Dry type	Fibrotic type
Exudative high attenuation ascites (HU 20-45), which may be free or loculated	Caseous mesenteric lymphadenopathy and fibrous adhesions with thickened, 'cake-like' omentum	Omental 'cake-like' mass with fixed bowel loops. Matted loops and mesentery with loculated ascites
On ultrasound fluid with internal echoes is seen		

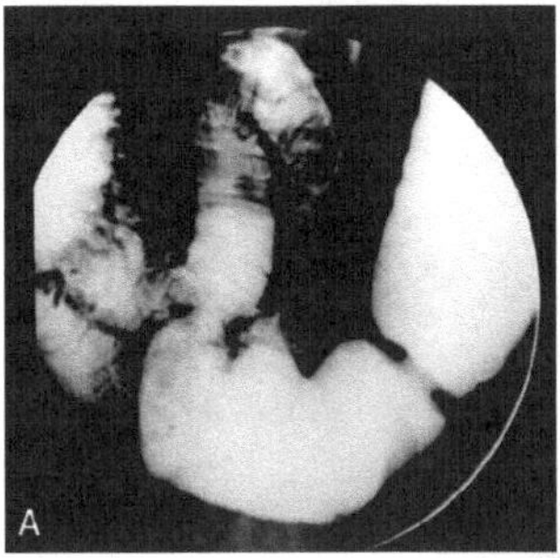

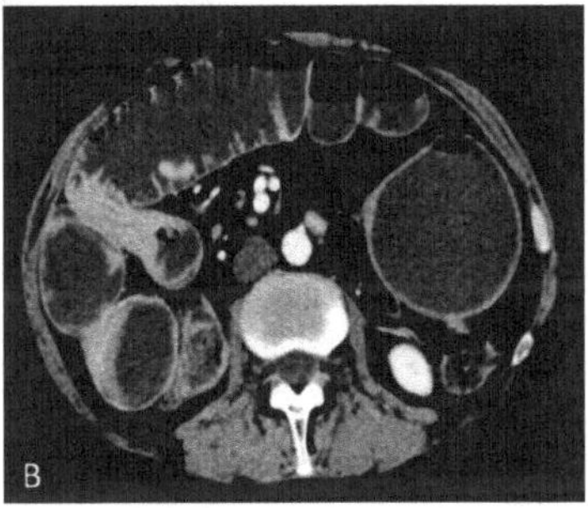

Figure 4.11: (A) BMFT examination study showing stricture with proximal dilatation of small bowel loops suggestive of tubercular stricture (B) Axial CT enterography study showing stricture with dilated bowel loops

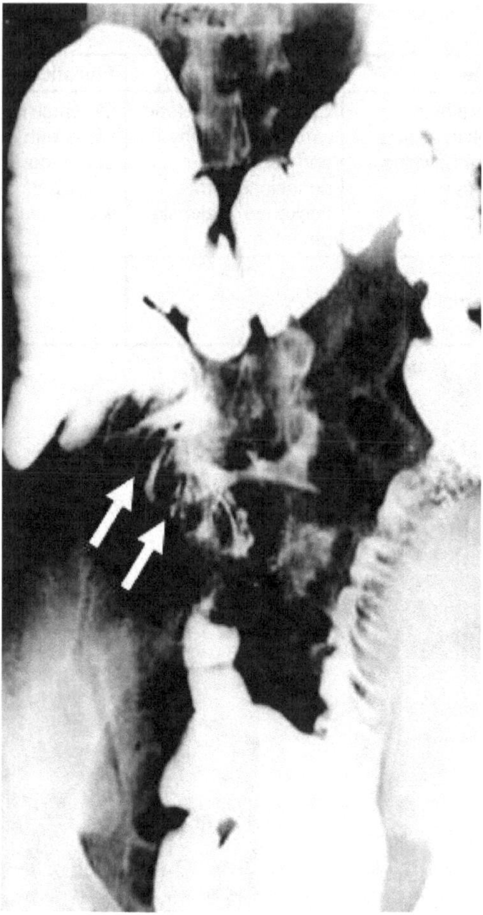

Figure 4.12: Barium meal follow through examination showing pulled up contracted cecum with hanging of terminal ileum giving a goose-neck appearance in a case of ileocecal tuberculosis

ANORECTAL MALFORMATIONS

Clinical Evaluation

Females	Males
One orifice – Common cloaca for urethra, vagina and rectum	Check the perineum whether external orifice is present or absent
Two orifices – One is urethral and other is vaginal orifice. In this case meconium is passed through the vaginal orifice since usually it is associated with recto-vaginal fistula	Absent external orifice→ urine is examined next for meconium→if meconium present then colostomy required and if meconium absent an invertogram is done to detect the level of anomaly
Three orifices – One is of urethra, other is vaginal orifice. Third orifice is of the bowel which can open at its normal site or may have a fistulous communication	

Colostomy is required in all cases except when three external orifices are seen in females and absence of meconium in urine in males but this varies from patient to patient.

Wingspread Classification of Anorectal Anomalies

Level	Male	Female
High Anomalies	1. Anorectal agenesis a. Without fistula b. With rectoprostatic urethral fistula 2. Rectal atresia	1. Anorectal agenesis a. Without fistula b. With rectovaginal fistula 2. Rectal atresia
Intermediate Anomalies	1. Anal agenesis without fistula 2. Rectobulbar urethral fistula	1. Anal agenesis without fistula 2. Rectovaginal fistula 3. Rectovestibular fistula
Low Anomalies	1. Anocutaneous fistula 2. Anal stenosis	1. Anovestibular fistula 2. Anocutaneous fistula 3. Anal stenosis
Cloacal Anomalies	Rare	Rare

Investigations: 1. Invertography 2. Contrast study 3. Ultrasound 4. MRI.

Invertography

Baby held upside down for 3 minutes, and strict lateral view is taken with thighs flexed at hip, and beam centered at greater trochanter. Barium paste or a marker is placed at anal dimple or natal cleft. An adequately taken invertogram is characterized by superimposed ischial bones and well-distended terminal blind bowel pouch.

The purpose of invertogram is to identify the relationship of blind pouch with levator ani muscle complex. For this purpose three lines are drawn: (i) pubococcygeal (PC) line (ii) ischial (I) line and (iii) anal pit line. If the gas bubble in the blind pouch is above the PC line, it is a high anomaly, if it is between PC and I line, it is an intermediate anomaly and if the gas bubble is below I line, it is classified as low anomaly.

Prone cross-table lateral view can also be done for this purpose if invertogram is not possible.

Contrast study: It is done to confirm the level of blind pouch and document presence or absence of fistula.

MRI: Better delineation of pelvic anatomy and measure the thickness of pelvic muscles.

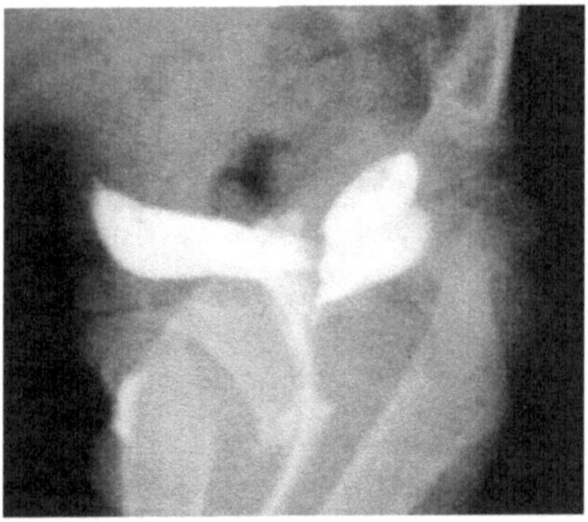

Figure 4.13: Colostography study showing opacification of urinary bladder, vagina, rectum and a common channel in a case of cloacal malformation

HIRSCHSPRUNG'S DISEASE

It is divided into 4 types according to the length of the aganglionic segment:

Short segment disease: 75% (rectal and distal sigmoid colonic involvement only).

Long segment: 15% (typically extends to splenic flexure / transverse colon).

Total colonic aganglionosis: 2 - 13% (also known as Zuezler-Wilson syndrome).

Ultrashort segment disease: 3 - 4 cm of internal anal sphincter only.

Imaging Findings

Plain film reveals dilated colon proximal to the aganglionic segment with small gas-filled rectum.

Radiological diagnosis is made with certainty after identifying the transition zone in a contrast enema study. Barium enema is performed after inserting a straight-tipped catheter just beyond the anal sphincter. Barium contrast should be prepared with normal saline to avoid possibility of water absorption from large surface area of dilated colon. The procedure should be stopped once the transition zone is identified.

The transition zone is a funnel-shaped zone of aganglionosis, is of small calibre with proximal dilatation. Fasciculation / saw-tooth irregularity of the aganglionic segment is frequently seen.

The rectosigmoid index can be used when the disease is confined to the rectum. If the sigmoid colon is more dilated than rectum (R/S index < 1), it is considered abnormal. This ratio is better estimated in early filling views.

Delayed radiographs taken after 24 hours is a must and shows prolonged retention of barium, which is a strong indicator of Hirschsprung's disease.

Difference between Hirschsprung's disease and small left colon syndrome

Hirschsprung's Disease	Small Left Colon Syndrome
Transition zone usually at rectosigmoid	Sudden change in calibre at splenic flexure
Funnel-shaped gradual tapering of transition zone	Abrupt change in calibre
Aganglionic segment of normal calibre	Entire left colon smaller in calibre
Rectum is of uniform calibre to the anus	Rectum is dilated

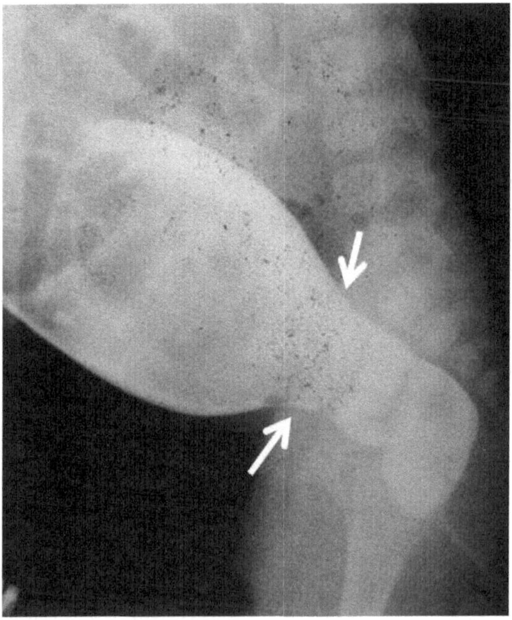

Figure 4.14: Contrast enema study in a case of Hirschsprung's disease showing funnel-shaped transition zone (arrow) with dilatation of proximal colon

NECROTISING ENTEROCOLITIS

Necrotising enterocolitis (NEC) is the most common acquired, life-threatening gastrointestinal condition affecting predominantly premature neonates. Its overall incidence is ~1 in 1000 live births and as high as 20% in extremely low birth weight infants (< 1000 g) and in infants of less than 28 weeks of gestational age. NEC usually develops 2 - 3 days following birth, with 90% developing within the first 10 days of life. Risk factors for NEC are prematurity, congenital heart disease, perinatal asphyxia, patent ductus arteriosus, indomethacin therapy, and decreased umbilical flow in utero.

Modified Bell's staging used for staging NEC classifies NEC into three stages.

Stage I–Clinical signs of apnea, bradycardia, lethargy, mild abdominal distension with or without blood in stools. Radiologically, abdominal radiographs are normal or may show mild ileus.

Stage II–Above signs plus mild thrombocytopenia, mild metabolic acidosis, absent bowel sounds, abdominal tenderness and abdominal cellulitis. Radiologically, this stage is characterized by ileus, pneumatosis intestinalis and portal venous gas.

Stage III–Above signs plus hypotension, respiratory acidosis, bradycardia, metabolic acidosis, DIC and neutropenia. Radiologically, pneumoperitoneum and ascites is seen.

Ominous signs in abdominal radiographs are persistence of dilatation, change other than in the normal direction, change from generalized to localized dilatation and fixed appearance of loops. The disappearance of intramural gas and portal venous gas is not always associated with clinical improvement, and these are thus poor indicators of progress.

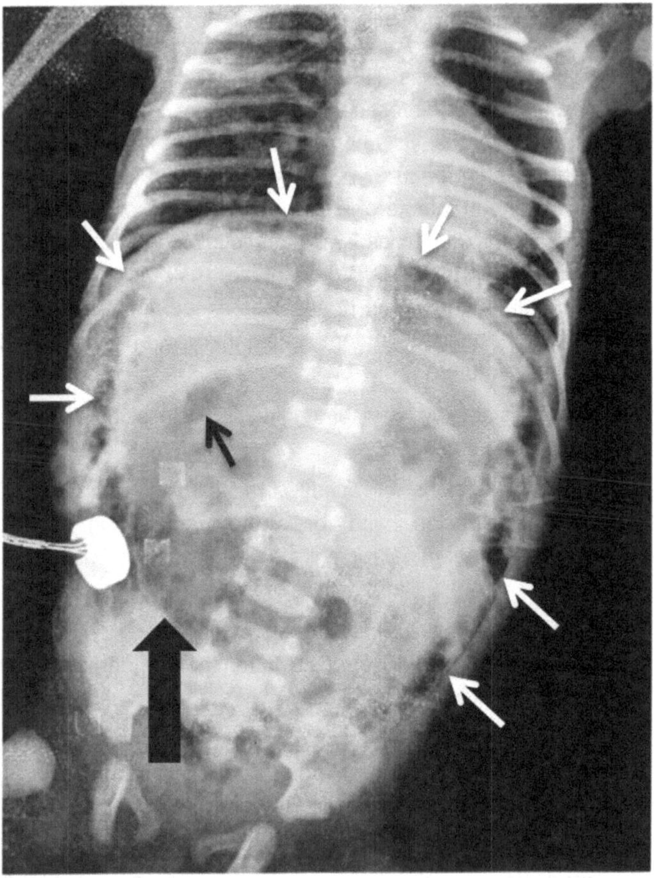

Figure 4.15: Supine abdomen radiograph of the child showing pneumoperitoneum–'Football sign' (white arrows), localised fixed mosaic appearance of bowel loops in right iliac fossa (black arrowhead) and hepatic-portal venous gas (black arrow)

CHOLEDOCHAL CYST

Types: Todani's classification

Type IA – Cystic dilatation of extrahepatic bile duct.

Type IB – Focal segmental dilatation.

Type IC – Fusiform dilatation.

Type II – Eccentric dilatation referred to as Choledochal diverticulum.

Type III – Choledochocele–Focal dilatation of intraduodenal portion of CBD.

Type IVA – Intahepatic and extrahepatic cysts.

Type IVB – Multiple cystic dilatations of extrahepatic ducts.

Type V – Caroli's disease (cystic dilatation of intrahepatic bile ducts).

Imaging Findings:

MRCP is the modality of choice.

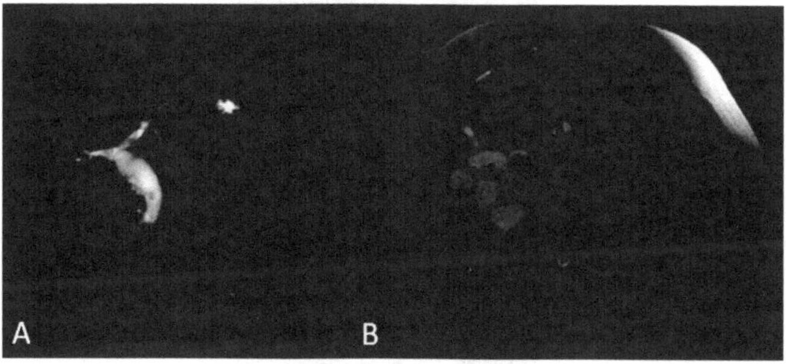

Figure 4.16: (A) Coronal T2 MRCP image showing fusiform dilatation of extrahepatic duct in a case of choledochal cyst Type I (B) Axial T2-weighted image showing Type V choledochal cyst with intraductal calculi

BILIARY ATRESIA

Imaging Findings

Ultrasonography

Gallbladder ghost triad: Triad of gallbladder length less than 19 mm, irregular or lobular contour and lack of smooth/complete echogenic mucosal lining with an indistinct wall.

Triangular cord sign: Echogenic triangular fibrotic tissue just cranial to the bifurcation of portal vein (thickness of echogenic anterior wall of right portal vein more than 4 mm).

Enlarged hepatic artery calibre: Diameter of > 1.5 mm at the level of proximal right hepatic artery or a hepatic artery diameter to portal vein diameter ratio of 0.45.

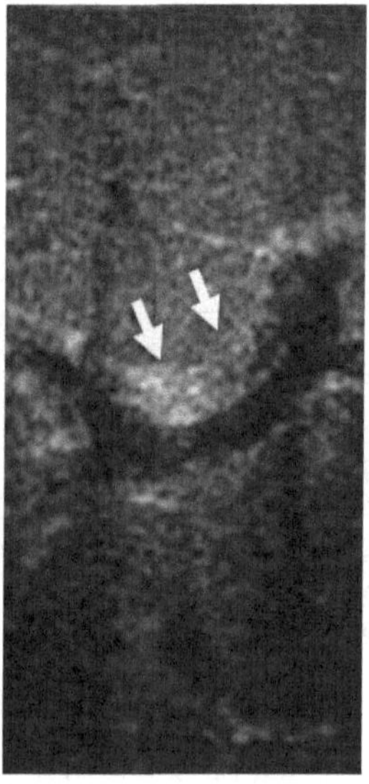

Figure 4.17: Ultrasound in a case of biliary atresia showing increased periportal echogenicity (arrows) suggestive of triangular cord sign

PORTAL HYPERTENSION

Causes

Pre Sinusoidal	Sinusoidal	Post Sinusoidal
Portal vein thrombosis	Cirrhosis	Budd-Chiari syndrome
Extrinsic compression of portal vein		Hepatic veno-occlusive disease
Schistosomiasis		Right heart failure

Imaging Findings

Ultrasound

Dilated portal vein > 13 mm, biphasic or reverse flow in portal vein in late stages and recanalisation of paraumbilical vein is pathognomic, splenomegaly, ascites and portal-systemic collateral pathways (collateral vessels/varices).

Also cause of portal hypertension is often identified.

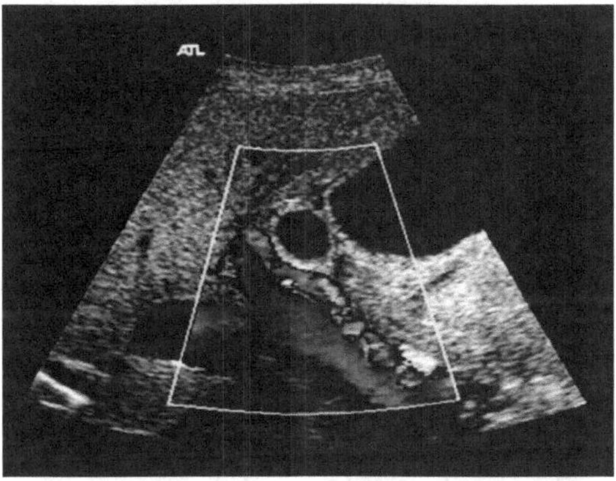

Figure 4.18: Doppler ultrasound image showing dilated portal vein with flow reversal in portal vein in a case of portal hypertension. Flow reversal is depicted by different color filling in hepatic artery and portal vein

LIVER ABSCESS

Plain Film

Indirect signs are gas within the abscess or biliary tree (pneumobilia) or beneath the diaphragm, right sided pleural effusion, calcification (hydatid cyst).

Ultrasound

Hypo or hyperechoic lesions with thick-irregular walls and absent of central vascularity.

CT

Appear as peripherally enhancing, centrally low density lesions. Occasionally in non-liquefied stage, they appear solid. Gas may be present. Segmental perfusion abnormalities, with early enhancement may be seen.

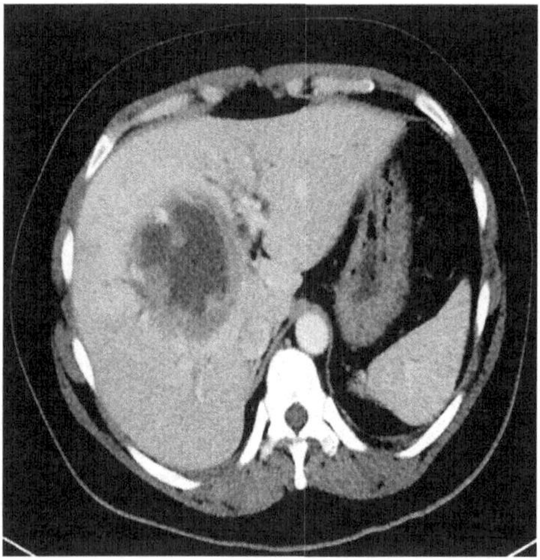

Figure 4.19: Axial contrast CT image showing hypodense liver abscess in right lobe of liver

MRI

Hypointense on T1 and Hyperintense on T2, shows diffusion restriction.

Bacterial and fungal abscesses are often multiple, whereas amoebic abscesses are more frequently single. Amoebic abscesses are more common in a sub-diaphragmatic location and are more likely to spread through the diaphragm and into the chest.

HYDATID CYST LIVER

Agents: Echinococcus granulosus and Echinococcus alveolaris.

CT: Fluid density cyst, with frequent peripheral focal areas of calcification. Septation, membranes and daughter cysts may be visualised.

MRI: Low signal on T1, mixed high signal on T2 depending on the cellular debris, septae and daughter cysts and on post-contrast scans, the walls and septae show enhancement.

Complications: Rupture into the biliary tree, peritoneal space, blood stream.

World Health Organization 2001 Classification of Hepatic Hydatid Cysts

CL - Unilocular anechoic cystic lesion without any internal echoes and septations.

CE 1 - Uniformly anechoic cyst with fine echoes settled in it representing hydatid sand.

CE 2 - Active stage. Cyst with multiple septations giving it multivesicular appearance or rossette appearance or honey-comb appearance with unilocular mother cyst.

CE 3 - Unilocular cyst with daughter cysts with detached laminated membranes appearing as water lily sign.

CE 4 - Mixed hypo and hyperechoic contents with absent daughter cysts, these contents give an appearance of ball of wool sign indicating the degenerative nature of the cyst.

CE 5 - Inactive stage. Arc like thick partially or completely calcified wall.

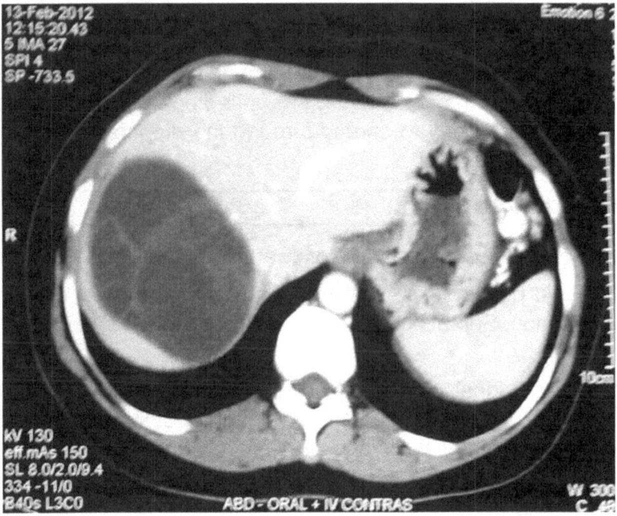

Figure 4.20: Axial contrast CT image showing classical hydatid cyst in liver

PEDIATRIC LIVER TUMORS

Malignant hepatic masses: Hepatoblastoma, hepatocellular carcinoma, fibrolamellar HCC, rhabdomyosarcoma, hepatic metastases.

Benign hepatic neoplasms: Infantile hemangioendothelioma, hemangioma, mesenchymal hamartoma, focal nodular hyperplasia, hepatic adenoma, peliosis hepatis.

Inflammatory lesions – Pyogenic hepatic abscess, amoebic hepatic abscess, fungal abscess, granulomatous lesions, hydatid cyst.

Simple cysts, polycystic liver disease, Caroli's disease.

WILMS' TUMOR AND NEUROBLASTOMA

Age: 1-5 years with a peak at 3 years of age.

Imaging

CT scan is more sensitive than ultrasound in identifying tumor extent, nodal and contralateral kidney involvement. On CT, Wilms' tumor is seen as a large, well defined heterogenously enhancing mass lesion arising from the kidneys. Calcification is very rare.

Differential diagnosis is neuroblastoma. Wilms' tumor arises from kidney whereas neuroblastoma displaces the kidney. Features in favour of Wilm's tumor are well defined margins, non-homogenous internal architecture with hemorrhage and necrosis and absence of calcification. Neuroblastoma shows evidence of ill-defined margins, tumor calcification, and tumor extension across midline, displacement and encasement of vascular structures. Encasement of aorta, paravertebral extension and invasion of spinal canal are highly predictive of neuroblastoma whereas tumor invasion of IVC and renal veins suggest Wilms' tumor.

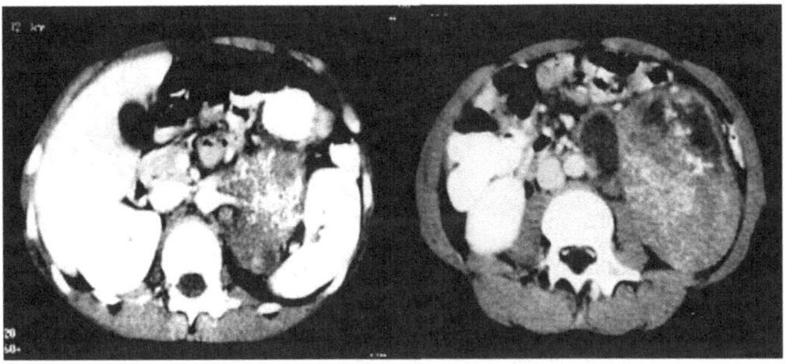

Figure 4.21: Axial contrast CT image showing left suprarenal mass with calcifications and encasement of vessels in a case of neuroblastoma

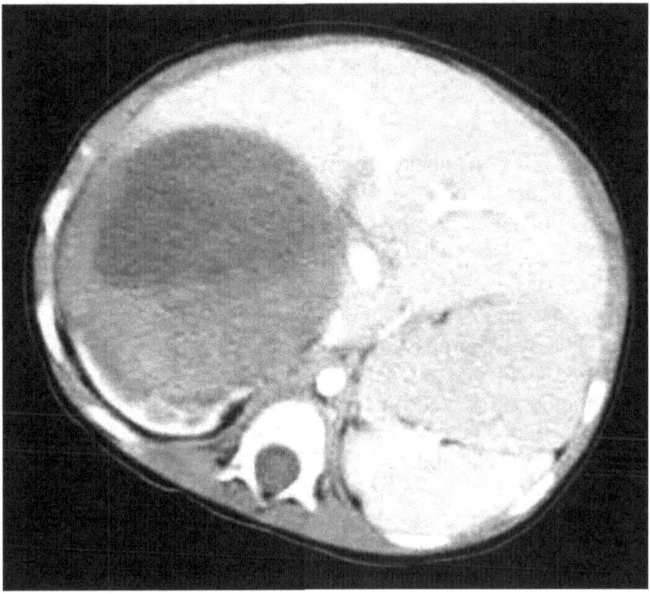

Figure 4.22: Axial contrast CT showing right renal mass in a case of Wilm's tumor in a child

PANCREATIC MASSES

Pancreatoblastoma.

Islet cell tumors.

Solid and papillary epithelial neoplasms (SPEN).

Mesenchymal tumors–lymphangioma, lipoma, teratoma, schwannoma, lymphoma.

Adenocarcinoma.

Pseudocysts.

Tuberculosis.

5

Chapter

Musculoskeletal System

RICKETS

Defect in mineralisation of normal osteoid tissue.

Imaging Findings

Classical changes occur at open growth plate.

The distal end of ulna is involved first as the distal ulnar growth plate grows more rapidly than the distal radius. Thus, changes in ulna are a more sensitive indicator at wrist joint.

Radiological Findings	Pathological Process
Osteopenia	Poor mineralisation
Widening of the growth plate earliest finding	Increase in cartilaginous cell mass
Irregular metaphyseal margins	Fraying and disorganization of spongy bone
Widening and cupping of metaphysis	Protrusion of the bulky mass of cartilaginous cells in the poorly mineralised metaphysis
Delayed appearance of ossificat-ion centres	Defective maturation and mineralisation
Rarefaction of shaft bones Thinned cortex	Loss of mineral content
Skull–Squared configuration known as craniotabes	Excess osteoid deposition in fronto parietal regions with posterior skull flattening
Long bones–Bowing deformities and rachitic rosary in ribs	Stress of weight bearing on weak bones

Contd.

Contd.

Spine–Scoliosis	Effects of weight bearing in weak bones
Pelvis–Triradiate configuration	Protrusion of hip and spine in weak pelvic bones
Fractures	Due to weak and poorly mineralised bones

Signs of Healing Rickets

Radiological evidence is usually seen after 2-3 weeks of therapy and takes around two months for complete recalcification.

- Reappearance of dense zone of provisional calcification – first sign; seen as a transverse line of increased density.
- Increase in cupping.
- Thickening of cortex.
- Reappearance/visualization of ossification centres due to recalcification.

Aetiological Consideration

Aetiology	Radiological Changes
Renal osteodystrophy	Combination of changes of rickets, secondary hyperparathyroidism and osteosclerosis Rugger jersey spine classical due to end plate bone deposition
Hereditary Vitamin D dependent rickets	Bone changes severe at presentation, rapidly progressive disease and usually associated with fractures
X-linked hypophosphatemia	Calcification and ossification of paravertebral, iliolumbar, sacroiliac ligaments and ligamentum flavum. Bony changes are of moderate grade and bowing of long bones is usually seen

Contd.

Contd.

Renal tubular acidosis (Type I)	Associated nephrocalcinosis/ nephrolithiasis
Tumor associated	Tumors associated with rickets are hemangiopericytoma, non-ossifying fibroma, giant cell tumor, hemangioma
Chemotherapeutic drugs	Particularly Ifosfamide

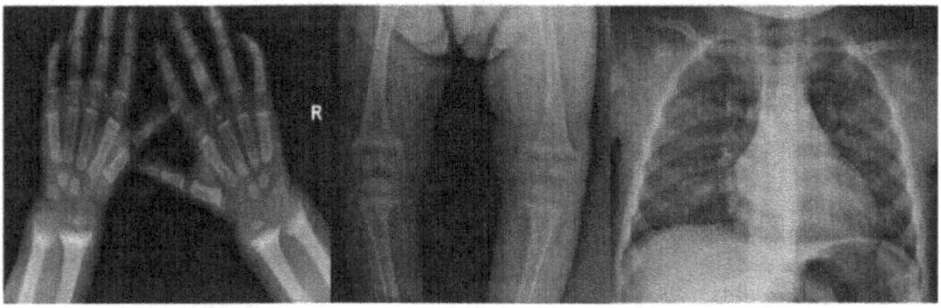

Figure 5.1: Radiograph of wrist, knee joint showing changes of nutritional rickets with osteopenia, cupping, fraying of metaphysis and chest X-ray showing evidence of rachitic rosary

SCURVY

Defect in osteoid formation due to long-term deficiency of Vitamin C. Rare before 6 months of age.

Imaging Findings:

- Osteoporosis.
- White line of Frankel – dense line at growing metaphysis at the zone of provisional calcification.
- Trummerfeld zone – Radiolucent zone below the Frankel's line – due to defect in osteoid formation.
- Wimberger sign–Small, sharply marginated and sclerotic epiphysis.
- Pelkan's spur – Fracture of metaphysis at margins.
- Subperiosteal hemorrhages – Seen later as calcified soft tissues adjacent the long bones – Sign of healing scurvy.

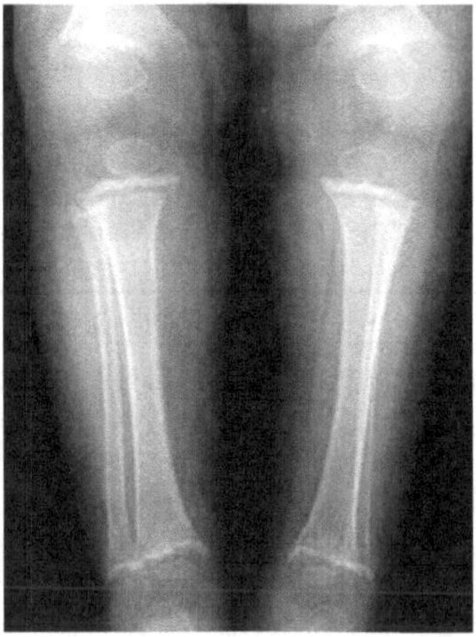

Figure 5.2: Radiograph of knee joint and legs in a child showing classical features of scurvy with evidence of osteopenia, thinned epiphyseal cortical rim, white line of Frankel and Trummerfeld zone

SALTER-HARRIS FRACTURES

Epiphyseal plate fractures–Can result in premature closure, limb shortening and abnormal growth. Typically occur in 10-15 years old child.

Imaging Findings

Salter-Harris Fracture Type	Radiological Changes
Type I – Good prognosis	Fracture plane through the growth plate
Type II – Good prognosis	Fracture plane through growth plate and metaphysis
Type III – Poor prognosis	Fracture plane through growth plate and epiphysis
Type IV – Poor prognosis	Fracture plane through growth plate, epiphysis and metaphysis
Type V – Worst prognosis	Crush injury of growth plate

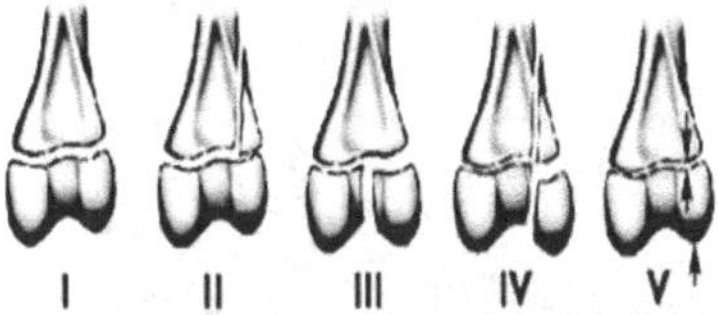

Figure 5.3: Figure showing different types of Salter-Harris fracture

Greenstick Fracture

Greenstick fractures are incomplete fractures of long bones and are usually seen in young children, more commonly less than 10 years of age. They are commonly mid-diaphyseal, affecting the forearm and lower leg.

X-Ray reveals fracture which is mid-diaphyseal, shows angulation with cortical breech of only one side of the bone.

Torus fractures (also known as buckle fractures) are incomplete fractures of the shaft of a long bone that is characterised by bulging of the cortex. On X-ray, distinct fracture lines are not seen, subtle deformity or buckle of the cortex may be evident and in some cases, angulation is the only diagnostic clue.

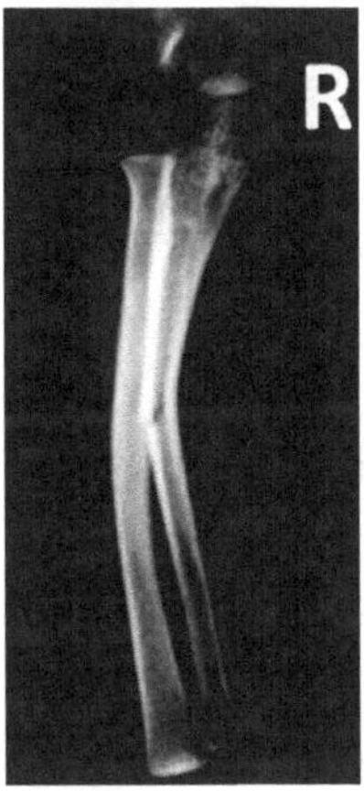

Figure 5.4: Radiograph of the right forearm showing greenstick fracture

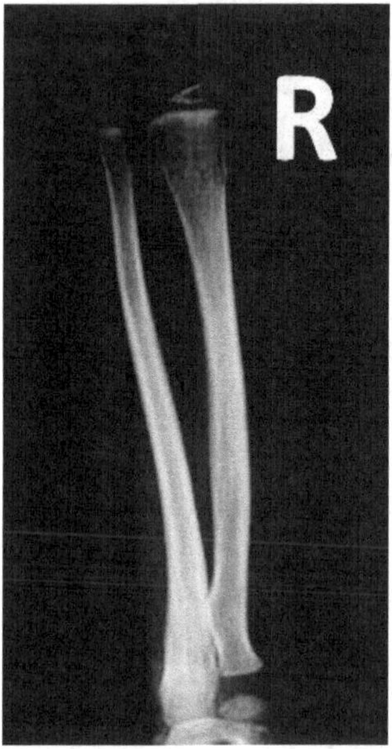

Figure 5.5: Radiograph of the right forearm showing torus fracture involving lower end of radius

OSTEOGENESIS IMPERFECTA

Imaging Findings

- Decrease in bony density.
- Thin gracile bones – brittle bones.
- Short thick limbs.
- Old healed fractures with mild residual deformity.
- Femoral fractures with excessive callus formation.
- Metaphyseal popcorn calcification.
- Platyspondyly.

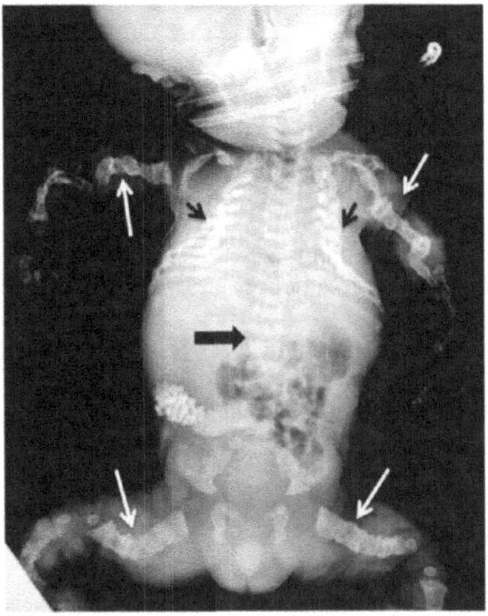

Figure 5.6: Infantogram showing generalized under mineralisation and evidence of multiple fractures. The ribs show continuous beading (black arrows). All long bones are short and broad with crumpled shafts (white arrows). Also there is evidence of bell-shaped chest with platyspondyly (arrowhead)

MUCOPOLYSACCHARIDOSES

Imaging Findings

MPS I Hurler Disease (Gargoylism)	MPS IV Morquio Disease
Clinical Features: Begins in early childhood Skeletal deformity Hepatosplenomegaly Corneal clouding Mentally challenged Mitral insufficiency	**Clinical Features:** Normal intelligence Joint laxity Knock knees Short stature

Contd.

Contd.

Premature closure–sagittal suture Clavical bones–thick Sella turcica – shalllow, elongated– 'J' shaped Mandible – short and broad Stylohyoid ligament calcification Proximal metacarpal pointing Widened metacarpal, proximal or middle phalanx Distal radius and ulna angulated Small irregular carpal bones Ribs–narrow at vertebral end and blunt Anteriorly–oar shaped Characteristic superior notching (inferior beaking) Small L1 vertebra Gibbus Intervertebral discs are normal Flared small iliac wings with inferior tapering Steep acetabular roofs Coxa valga	Hypoplastic odontoid Atlanto-axial dislocation Occipitalisation arch of atlas Broad ribs–not oar shaped Sternal protrusion Dysplastic femoral head epiphysis Central beaking

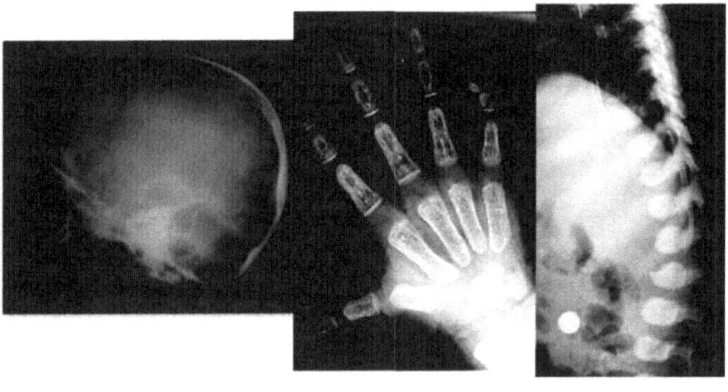

Figure 5.7: Skull radiograph lateral view showing J-shaped sella in a case of mucopolysaccharidosis. Radiograph of hands and spine showing osteopenia, proximal pointing of metacarpals and inferior beaking in a case of Hurler's syndrome

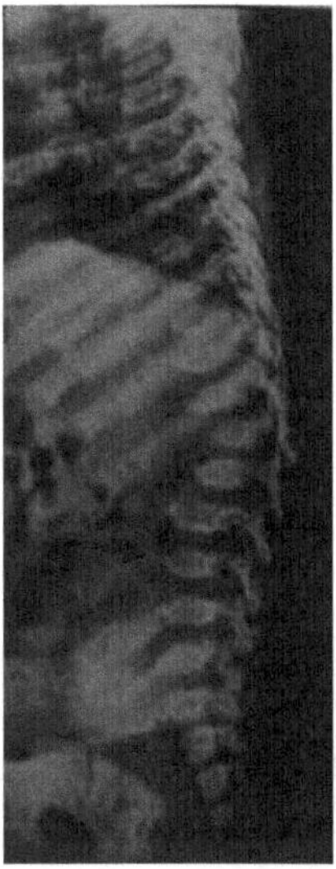

Figure 5.8: Radiograph of spine showing central beaking in a case of Morquio syndrome

ACHONDROPLASIA

Clinical Features

Short limb rhizomelic dwarfness.

Head large in relation to body.

Saddle shaped nose.

Prominent buttocks in infancy.

Trident shaped hands.

Normal intelligence.

Imaging Findings

Spine: Pedicles short and thick, lumbar canal stenosis, posterior scalloping.

Skull: Large cranial vault with small skull base, prominent forehead with depressed nasal bridge, foramen magnum narrowed.

Hands: Short and broad metacarpals and phalanges, trident hand.

Pelvis: Champagne-glass pelvis, squared iliac wings, flat acetabulae.

Long bones: Short broad tibiae, fibulae are relatively longer, epiphyses have a v-shaped configuration.

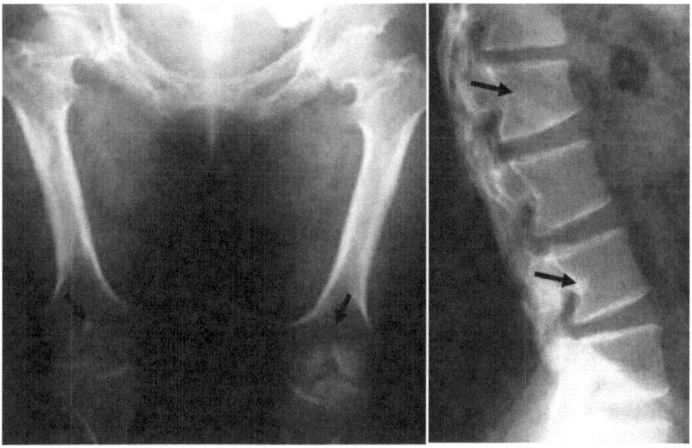

Figure 5.9: Radiograph of pelvis and spine showing v-shaped configuration of epiphysis, posterior scalloping of vertebrae and lumbar canal stenosis in a case of achondroplasia

ASPHYXIATING THORACIC DYSTROPHY (JEUNE'S SYNDROME)

Imaging Findings

High handle bar appearance of clavicles.

Narrow thorax.

Short horizontal ribs.

Wide irregular costochondral junctions.

Trident appearance of pelvis.

Metaphyseal irregularity.

Skull and spine are normal.

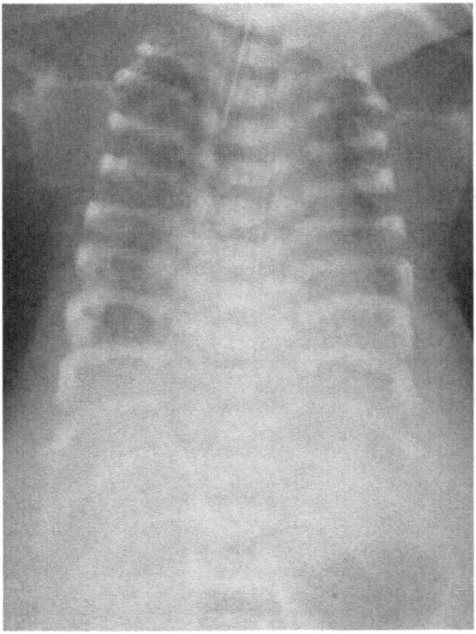

Figure 5.10: Radiograph of chest showing narrow bell shaped chest in a case of Jeune's syndrome

OSTEOPETROSIS

Clinical Features

Two forms: Lethal autosomal recessive form and milder autosomal dominant form.

Pancytopenia.

Hepatosplenomegaly.

Cranial nerve palsies.

Recurrent infection, hemorrhage.

Imaging Findings

Uniform sclerosis of the calvaria and skull base.

Extensive sclerosis of the different bony elements of the thoracic cage (ribs, clavicles).

Loss of corticomedullary differentiation.

Alternate areas of mature bone and sclerotic osseous tissue give a "bone within bone" appearance.

Sandwich vertebrae/Rugger-Jersey spine.

Presence of 'endobones' within the iliac wings, acetabuli, sacrum and pubic bones.

Erlenmeyer flask deformity.

Metaphyseal bands.

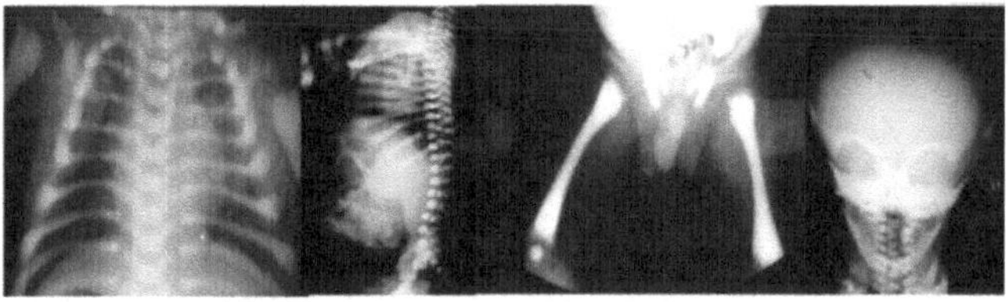

Figure 5.11: Series of radiographs of chest, spine, femora and skull showing increased density of bones in a case of osteopetrosis

DOWN'S SYNDROME

Imaging Findings

Musculoskeletal system: Eleven ribs, hyper-segmented sternum, joint laxity/dislocation(s), developmental dysplasia of the hip (DDH), atlanto-axial subluxation and atlanto-occipital instability, hypoplastic posterior arch of C1.

Gastrointestinal system: Duodenal atresia, anal atresia, Hirschsprung's disease, omphalocoele.

Respiratory system: Pulmonary hypoplasia, pulmonary cysts, pig bronchus.

Cardiovascular system: Congenital heart diseases like atrioventricular septal defect (AVSD), atrial septal defect (ASD), ventricular septal defect (VSD).

SEPTIC ARTHRITIS

Imaging Findings

Plain film: Destruction of subchondral bone on both sides of a joint; juxta-articular osteoporosis; joint effusion may be seen.

Ultrasound: Joint effusion (with internal echoes).

CT: Joint effusion and bone erosions around the joint; fat-fluid level can be a specific sign in the absence of trauma.

MRI: Synovial enhancement; perisynovial edema.

Transient synovitis: Older than 4 years of age, no history of fever.

Septic arthritis: Younger than 4 years, history of fever and joint effusion.

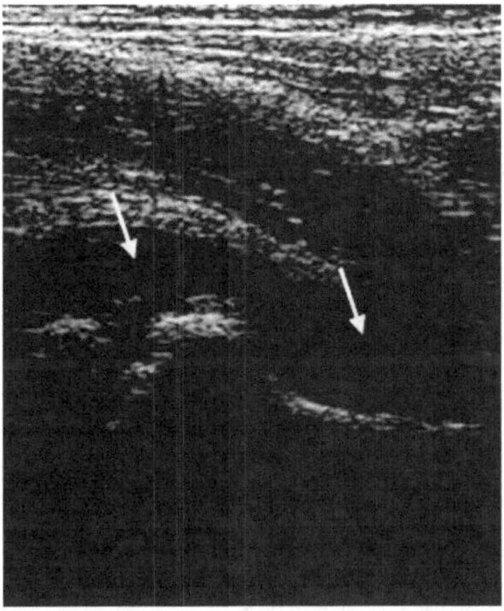

Figure 5.12: Ultrasound of hip joint showing joint effusion with internal echoes in a case of septic arthritis of hip

OSTEOMYELITIS

Bony inflammation that is almost always due to infection, typically bacterial.

Imaging Features

Plain film: Early findings may be subtle, and changes may not be obvious until 5 to 7 days in children and 10 to 14 days in adults.

- Regional osteopenia.
- Periosteal reaction/thickening–variable and may appear aggressive including formation of a Codman's triangle.
- Focal lucencies.
- Endosteal scalloping.
- Loss of bony trabecular architecture.
- New bone apposition.
- Eventual peripheral sclerosis.

The earliest changes are seen in adjacent soft tissues +/- muscle outlines with swelling and loss or blurring of normal fat planes. An effusion may be seen in an adjacent joint.

In chronic or untreated cases eventual formation of a sequestrum, involucrum or cloaca may be seen.

CT and MRI: CT is superior to both MRI and plain film in depicting the bony margins and identifying a sequestrum or involucrum. MRI is most sensitive and specific and is able to identify soft-tissue/joint complications.

Ultrasound: Mainly to look for soft tissue abscesses, cellulitis, sub periosteal collections and joint effusion.

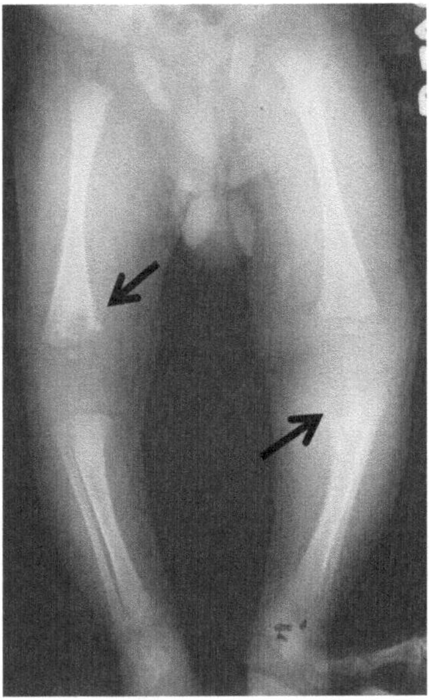

Figure 5.13: Radiograph of both knees showing pyogenic osteomyelitis in the form of lytic lesions (arrow)

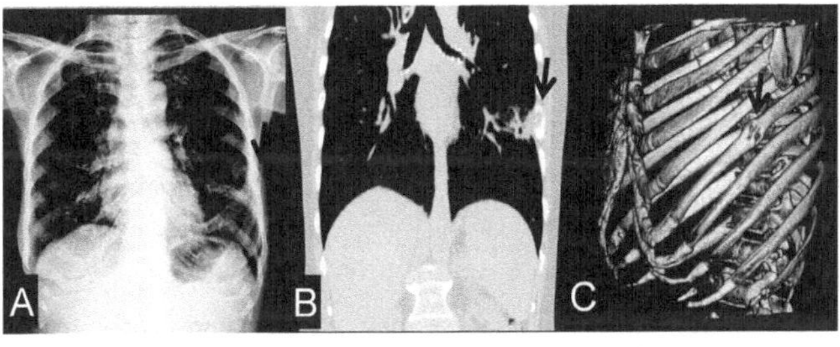

Figure 5.14: (A) Chest radiograph (B) Coronal reformatted CT scan (C) VR image showing cavitating lung lesion on left side with destruction of rib in a case of tubercular osteomyelitis

LEAD POISONING

Imaging Findings

Plain film.

Dense metaphyseal bands.

Bone within bone appearance may be seen.

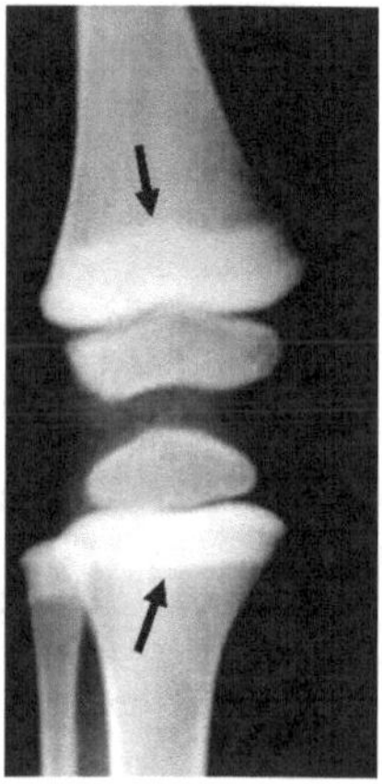

Figure 5.15: Radiograph of knee joint showing dense metaphyseal bands in a case of lead poisoning

HYPOTHYROIDISM

X-ray Manifestations

- Delayed skeletal maturation (bone age lagging behind chronological age).
- Wormian bones.
- Irregular and late appearance of epiphyses (epiphyseal dysgenesis).
- Delayed closure of epiphyseal plates.
- Sella may be small or large.

- Underdeveloped paranasal sinuses.
- Bullet shaped vertebrae.
- Metaphyseal bands.
- Coxa vara deformity in pelvis.
- Slipped capital femoral epiphyses.

SLIPPED CAPITAL FEMORAL EPIPHYSES

Conditions that may predispose a child to a SCFE are:

Hypothyroidism.

Hypopituitarism.

Hyperparathyroidism.

X-Ray Findings

Slip occurs mostly in posteromedial direction which is seen on frog-leg lateral view.

Normally, a line drawn tangential to the lateral border of the femoral neck intercepts the epiphyseal ossification centre so that a small portion of the head remains lateral to this line.

In slipped capital femoral epiphyses (SCFE), no femoral head ossification centre is seen lateral to the line. On an AP radiograph, there may be mild widening, lucency and irregularity of the physis.

Ultrasound

Findings are non-specific and may show joint effusion.

MRI

Physeal widening is seen on T1 weighted images; synovitis and marrow edema better seen on T2 weighted images.

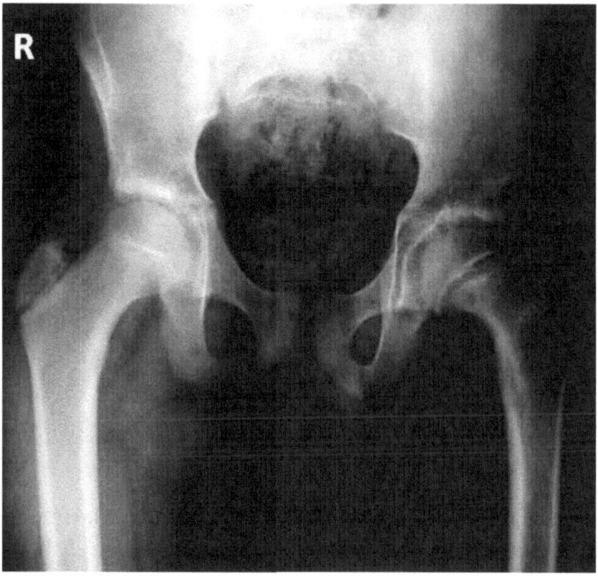

Figure 5.16: Radiograph of pelvis in a child presenting with limping showing slipped capital femoral epiphysis on the left side

DEVELOPMENTAL DYSPLASIA OF HIP

X-Ray Findings

Look for symmetry of femoral epiphyses. Delayed ossification and asymmetry is a sign of DDH.

Hilgenreiner's line: Hilgenreiner's line is drawn horizontally through the superior aspect of both triradiate cartilages. It should be horizontal, but is mainly used as a reference for Perkin's line and measurement of the acetabular angle.

Perkin's line: Perkin's line is drawn perpendicular to Hilgenreiner's line, intersecting the lateral most aspect of the acetabular roof. The upper femoral epiphysis should be seen in the inferomedial quadrant (i.e. below Hilgenreiner's line and medial to Perkin's line).

Acetabular angle: The acetabular angle is formed by the intersection between a line drawn tangential to the acetabular roof and Hilgenreiner's line, forming an acute angle. It should be approximately 30 degrees at birth and progressively reduce with maturation of the joint.

Shenton's line: Shenton's line is drawn along the inferior border of the superior pubic ramus and should continue laterally along the inferomedial aspect of the proximal femur as a smooth line. If there is superolateral migration of the proximal femur due to DDH then this line will be discontinuous.

Ultrasound

Ultrasound is the test of choice in the infant (< 6 months) as the proximal femoral epiphysis has not yet significantly ossified. Additionally it has the advantage of being a real time dynamic examination allowing the stability of the hip to be assessed with stress views.

Alpha angle: Angle formed by the acetabular roof to the vertical cortex of the ilium. This is a similar measurement as that of the acetabular angle. The normal value is greater than or equal to 60 degrees.

Beta angle: Angle formed between the vertical cortex of the ilium and the triangular labral fibrocartilage (echogenic triangle). The normal value is less than 77 degrees, but is only useful in assessing immature hips when combined with the alpha angle.

Bony coverage: The percentage of the femoral epiphysis covered by the acetabular roof. A value of greater than 58% is considered normal.

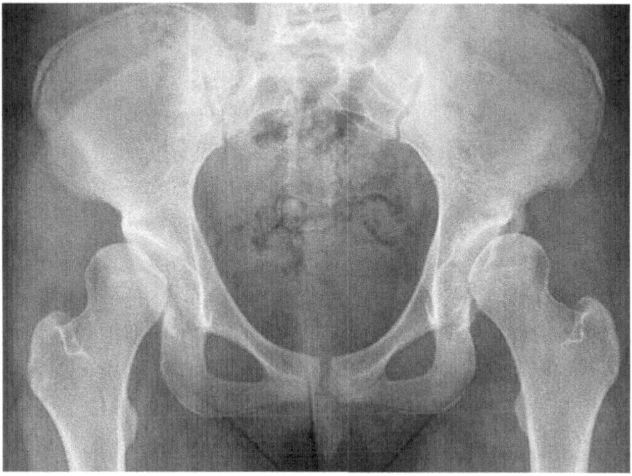

Figure 5.17: Radiograph of pelvis showing lack of femoral head coverage laterally and the break in Shenton's line in a case of bilateral DDH

SACRAL AGENESIS

Sacral agenesis is a rare and severe sacral developmental abnormality. It is a part of caudal regression syndrome.

Classification

Type I – Unilateral agenesis localised to sacrum or coccyx.

Type II – Partial agenesis with bilateral defects; the iliac bone articulates with S1, but the distal sacral elements fail to develop.

Type III – Total sacral agenesis; iliac bones articulate with the lowest lumbar element.

Type IV – Total sacral agenesis; iliac bones fuse posteriorly.

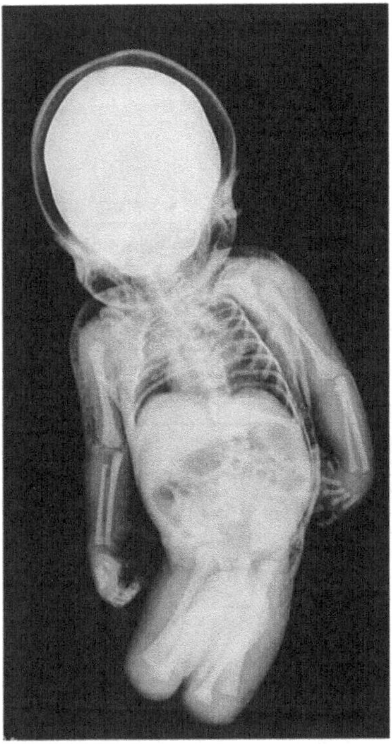

Figure 5.18: Postmortem infantogram showing multiple congenital anomalies, sacral agenesis and sirenomelia

BONE AGE ESTIMATION

The most common and widely accepted method for assessing skeletal age is to perform a plain film of the left hand and wrist.

Methods

1. Appearance and fusion of ossification centres.
2. Greulich and Pyle atlas method (G-P method).
3. Tanner and Whitehouse II method (TW2 method).

Different Radiographs are Required for Bone Age Depending upon Expected Age:

- PA radiograph of wrist and hand.
- Elbow, knee, shoulder.
- Pelvis AP for iliac crest.

Appearance and Fusion of Ossification Centres

Wrist-Capitate – 4 mths, Hamate – 4 mths, triquetral – 3 yrs, lunate – 4-5 yrs, trapezium – 6 yrs, trapezoid – 6 yrs, scaphoid – 6 yrs, pisiform – 11 yrs
Metacarpal heads – 2.5 yrs, fuse 20th yr
Base of proximal phalanges – 2.5 yrs, fuse 20th yr
Base of middle phalanges – 3 yrs, fuse 18-20 yrs
Base of distal phalanges – 3 yrs, fuse 18-20 yrs
Base of 1st metacarpal – 2.5 yrs, fuse 20th yr
Lower end of radius – 1-2 yrs, fuses 20th yr
Lower end of ulna – 5-8 yrs, fuses 20th yr
Lateral epicondyle – 10-12 yrs, fuse 17-18 yrs
Medial epicondyle – 5-8 yrs, fuse 17-18 yrs
Capitulum – 1-3 yrs, fuse 17-18 yrs
Head of radius – 5-6 yrs, fuse 16-19 yrs
Trochlea – 11th yr, fuse 18th yr
Olecranon – 10-13 yrs, fuse 16-20 yrs
Medial end of clavicle – 18-20 yrs, fuse 25th yr
Femoral head – 1st yr, fuse 18-20 yrs
Greater trochanter of femur – 3-5 yrs, fuse 18-20 yrs
Lesser trochanter of femur – 8-14 yrs, fuse 18-20 yrs
Femur and tibial epiphysis upper – At birth, fuse 20th yr
Upper end of fibula – 4th yr, fuse 25th yr
Iliac crest – Appear about puberty, fuse at 20-25 yrs
Foot – calcaneum, talus – 6th fetal mths, navicular -3-4yrs, cuboid at birth, lateral cuneiform 1 yr, middle cuneiform 3 yrs, medial cuneiform 3 yrs.

6

Chapter

Central Nervous System

NORMAL SKULL MEASUREMENTS

Cephalic Index: 75-85.

Head: Face ratio – 2.5:1.

Suture size: <2 mm after 3 years.

Thickness of outer table of skull – 1.5 mm.

Thickness of inner table of skull – 0.5 mm.

Basal Angle: 123-143 degrees; Angle greater than 143 degrees is platybasia.

Sella Dimensions: AP<17 mm; Depth<13 mm; Width- 10-15 mm

Carotid canal – 6.5 mm.

Internal acoustic meatus and optic foramen <7 mm.

Difference between two sides <2 mm.

Closure of posterior fontanelle – 1-3 months.

Closure of anterior fontanelle – last to close between 7-19 months.

Closure of sphenoidal fontanelle – At around 6 months of age.

Closure of mastoid fontanelle – 6-18 months.

CRANIOSYNOSTOSIS

Craniosynostosis refers to premature closure of the cranial sutures.

Examples:

Brachycephaly - Bicoronal and/or bilamboid sutures.

Scaphocephaly/Dolichocephaly - Sagittal suture.

Plagiocephaly - Unilateral coronal and lambdoid sutures.

Trigonocephaly - Metopic suture.

Pachycephaly - Lamdoid suture.

Oxycephaly/Turricephaly - Sagittal, coronal and lambdoid sutures (Tower like skull).

Clover leaf skull/Kleeblattschadel - Intrauterine sagittal, coronal, lambdoid sutures - Most severe.

Harlequin eye - Ipsilateral coronal suture.

Skull X-ray shows evidence of copper beaten skull: Copper beaten skull (also known as **beaten brass skull**) refers to the prominence of convolutional markings (gyral impressions on the inner table of the skull) seen throughout the skull vault. The appearance of copper beaten skull is associated with raised intracranial pressure in children. Convolutional markings may be normal, but are usually confined to the posterior part of the skull's inner table.

Conditions which may show evidence of copper beaten skull are:

- Craniosynostosis.
- Obstructive hydrocephalus.
- Hypophosphatasia.
- Intracranial masses.

Causes:

Syndromic–Apert's, Carpenter's, Pfeiffer's, Crouzon's syndrome.

Secondary–Metabolic(rickets,hyperthyroidism,hypophosphatasia); Inborn errors of metabolism (MPS), Thalassemia, Sickle cell anemia, Congenital brain malformations, Shunted hydrocephalus.

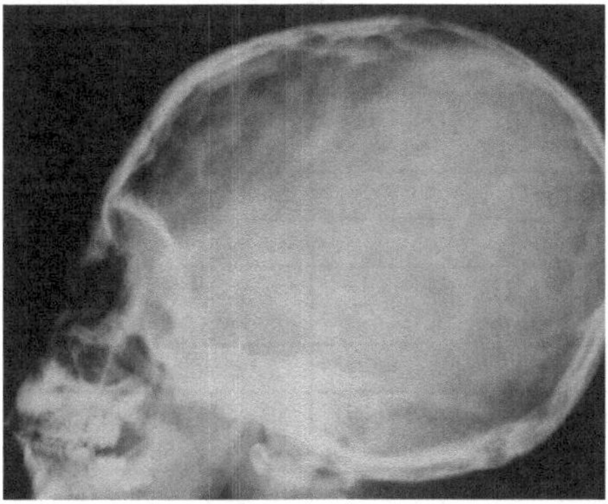

Figure 6.1: Skull radiograph lateral view showing copper beaten skull in a case of craniosynostosis

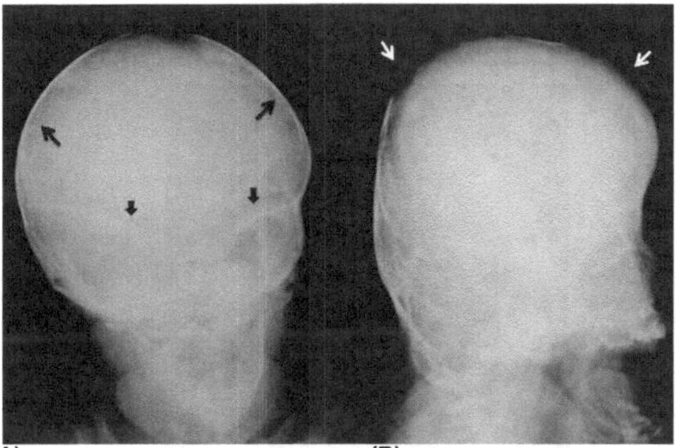

(A) (B)

Figure 6.2: Skull X-ray (A) AP view shows fusion of coronal sutures (arrows) and elevated superolateral angles of both orbits (arrow heads) giving the appearance of 'harlequin mask' (B) Lateral view shows classical turribrachycephalic skull (white arrows) in a case of Apert's syndrome

DIFFERENCE BETWEEN NEUROCYSTICERCOSIS AND TUBERCULOMA

Neurocysticercosis	**Tuberculoma**
Size less than 2 cm	Size more than 2 cm
Eccentric calcification	Central or target calcification
Fluid is cystic	Fluid is exudative/proteinaceous in nature
Less edema	More edema
Thin peripheral rim	Thick, irregular rim
Usually no evidence of meningitis	Other signs like meningitis, basal exudates
T2 hyperintensity	T2 hypointensity
MR Spectroscopy: Absent lipid peak	MR Spectroscopy: Lipid peak at 0.9,1.3,2.0 and 2.8 ppm
Eccentric scolex	No scolex
No conglomeration	Conglomerated lesions
Complications usually not seen	May be associated with complications like hydrocephalus, vasculitis and neuropathies

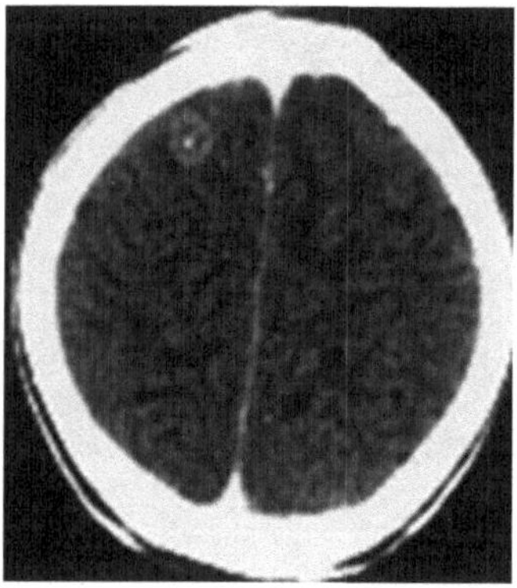

Figure 6.3: CECT head showing ring enhancing lesion in right frontal lobe with eccentric calcified scolex suggestive of neurocysticercosis

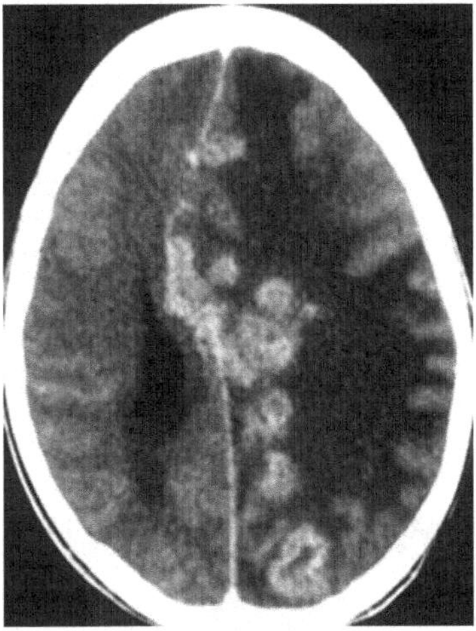

Figure 6.4: CECT head showing multiple ring enhancing lesions with moderate edema and midline shift in a case of multiple tuberculomas

DIFFERENTIATION BETWEEN ARTERIAL AND VENOUS INFARCT

Arterial Infarct	Venous Infarct
Confined to an arterial territory	Does not confine to a vascular territory
Not hemorrhagic initially but may show hemorrhagic transformation in subacute stage	Hemorrhagic
Grey-white matter involvement	Peripheral, heterogeneous and gyriform
Arterial thrombosis	Dural sinus thrombosis and deep cerebral venous thrombosis
Wedge shaped	Irregular in shape
Unilateral	May be bilateral
Isolated cortical edema uncommon	Cortical hemorrhages and edema common

Contd.

Contd.

Absent dense clot and empty delta sign	**Dense clot sign positive** – Direct visualization of a clot in the cerebral veins on a non-enhanced CT scan is known as the dense clot sign. **Empty delta sign positive** – The empty delta sign is a finding that is seen on a contrast enhanced CT (CECT). The sign consists of a triangular area of enhancement with a relatively low-attenuating centre, which is the thrombosed sinus. **Pseudodelta sign** – Sign seen on NCCT head in patients with subarachnoid or subdural hemorrhage.

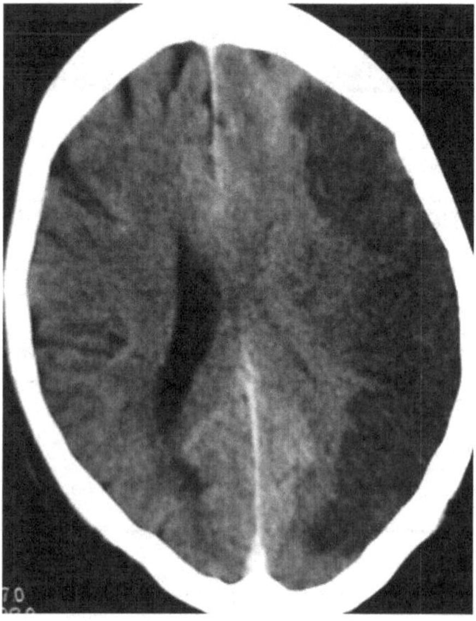

Figure 6.5: Axial non-contrast CT head showing wedge shaped hypodensity in left fronto-parieto-occipital region confined to an arterial territory suggestive of left MCA territory infarct

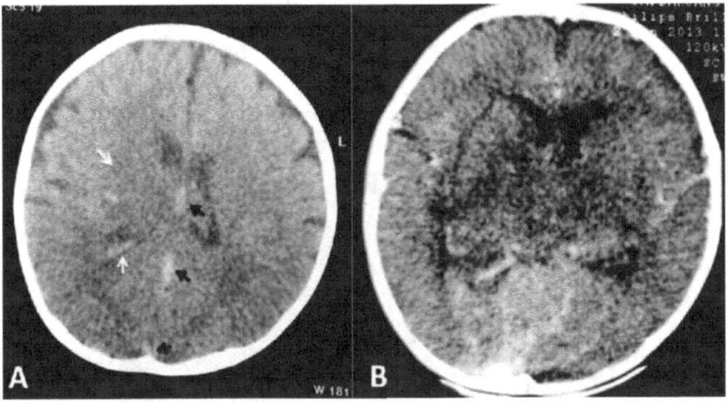

Figure 6.6: (A) Non-enhanced computed tomography (CT) head showing linear hyperdense cord sign involving the deep venous system (black arrows), hemorrhages and hypodense (white arrows) right thalamus and basal ganglia (B) Contrast-enhanced CT head showing hypodensity involving bilateral thalami and basal ganglia suggestive of deep venous system infarct

DIFFERENTIATION BETWEEN ACUTE, SUBACUTE AND CHRONIC INFARCT

Acute Infarct	**Subacute Infarct (<2 weeks)**	**Chronic Infarct (> 2 weeks)**
Hyperacute infarct (< 12 hours) Hyperdense MCA sign on NCCT head (due to acute intraluminal thrombus within MCA) Obscuration of lentiform nucleus ***Acute infarct (12-24 hours)*** Low density basal ganglia Loss of gray-white interface (Insular ribbon sign) Sulcal effacement	Increasing mass effect Wedge-shaped low density area Hemorrhagic transformation Gyral enhancement ***Fogging effect on MRI*** – Normal appearance on T2 weighted sequences, but shows enhancement on postcontrast T1 weighted sequences	Encephalo-malacic changes Volume loss Rarely calcification

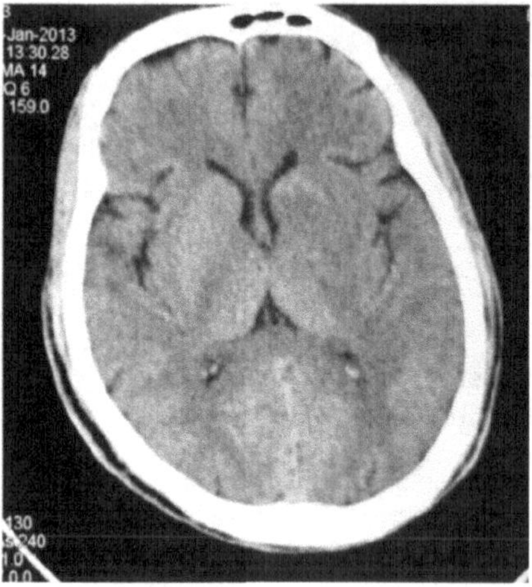

Figure 6.7: Axial non-contrast CT head scan showing low density left basal ganglia suggestive of acute infarct.

METABOLIC AND WHITE MATTER DISEASES OF THE BRAIN WITH IMAGING CHARACTERISTICS

Disorders that primarily affect the white matter (Leukodystrophies)
Metchromatic leukodystrophy – Near complete lack of myelination.
Krabbe disease–Hyperdense basal ganglia and thalami on NCCT; demyelination involving the periventricular and parieto-occipital white matter.
Adrenoleukodystrophy – Demyelination of occipital white matter (peritrigonal region) and splenium of corpus callosum.
Pelizaeus – Merzbacher disease – "tigroid or leopard-skin" pattern (demyelination of white matter with sparing of perivascular white matter).
Alexander disease – Macrocephaly; demyelination of frontal white matter.

Contd.

Contd.

Canavan disease – Macrocephaly; near complete lack of myelination with involvement of subcortical U-fibres. Phenylketonuria – Periventricular demyelination. Maple syrup urine disease – Demyelination of cerebellar white matter, dorsal brainstem. Homocystinuria–Arterial thromboembolic infarcts, venous thrombosis. Glutaric aciduria Type I – Batwing sign – dilatation of sylvian fissures.
Disorders affecting gray matter
Tay-Sachs disease – T2 hyperintensity in thalamus and basal ganglia; severe cortical atrophy. Hurler Syndrome – Gross meningeal thickening. Glycogen Storage diseases – Nonspecific cortical atrophy.
Disorders affecting both gray and white matter
Leigh disease – T2 hyperintensity in basal ganglia, periventricular white matter and periaqueductal gray matter; strokes. Zellweger syndrome–Heterotopia, pachygyria-polymicrogyria complex; markedly diminished white matter volume (hypomyelination).
Basal ganglia disorders
Huntington disease – Basal ganglia atrophy causing focal enlargement of frontal horns. Hallervorden-Spatz disease – Eye-of the tiger sign (T2 hyperintensity in medial part of globus pallidus and hypointensity in lateral part). Fahr disease – Calcifications in basal ganglia, centrum semiovale, dentate nuclei and subcortical white matter. Wilson disease – Giant panda sign seen in midbrain (T2 MR sequence showing hyperintensity in midbrain with sparing of red nucleus, superior colliculus, lateral part of pars reticulata).

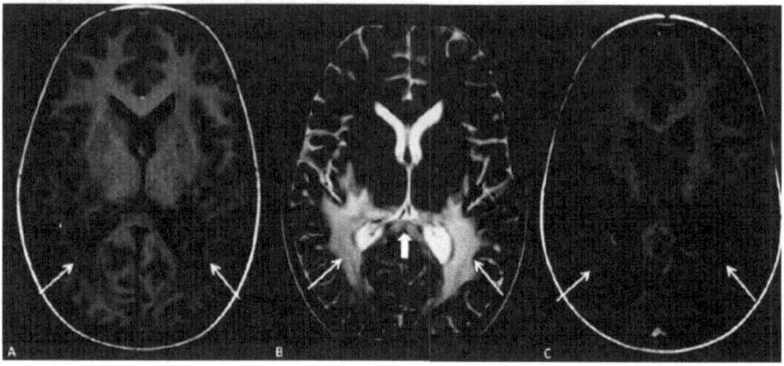

Figure 6.8: (A) Axial MR brain T1WI showing abnormal hypointense signal intensity involving peritrigonal region (arrows) (B) Axial MR brain T2WI showing abnormal hyperintense signal involving the peritrigonal region (arrows) and splenium of corpus callosum (arrowhead) (C) Axial MR brain T1 post-contrast image showing enhancement of the intermediate zone (arrows) in a case of Adrenoleukodystrophy

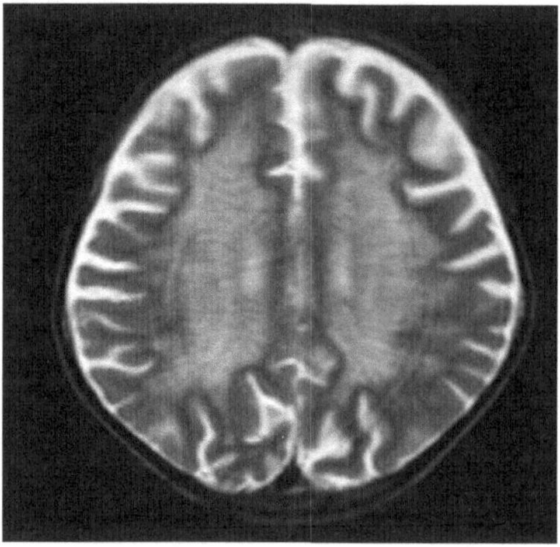

Figure 6.9: Axial T2-weighted MR image showing "tigroid or leopard-skin" pattern in a case of Pelizaeus–Merzbacher disease

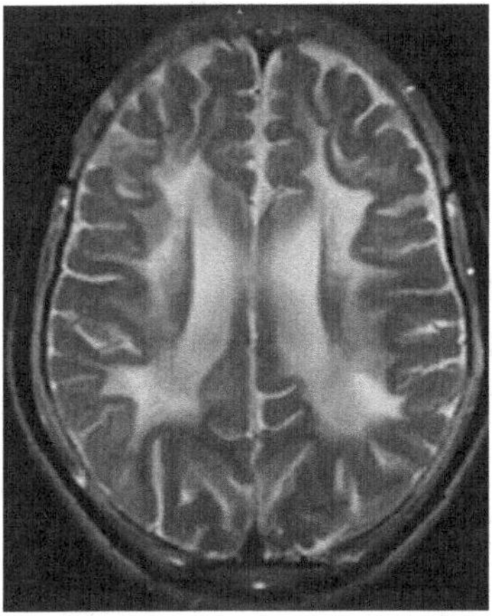

Figure 6.10: Axial T2-weighted MR image showing white matter hyper-intensity in periventricular white matter in a case of metachromatic leukodystrophy

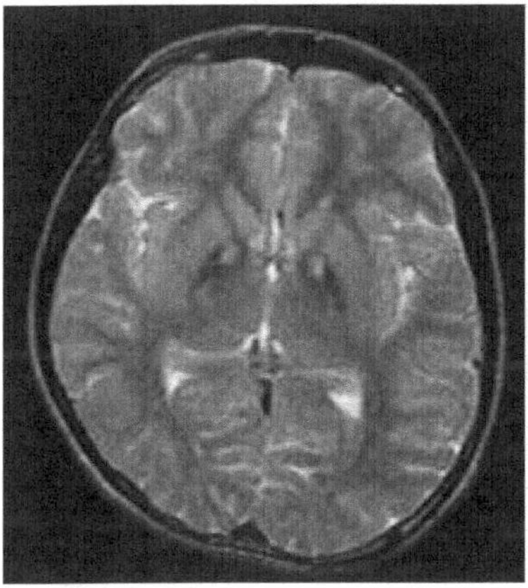

Figure 6.11: Axial T2-weighted MR image showing eye of the tiger sign in a case of Hallervorden-Spatz disease

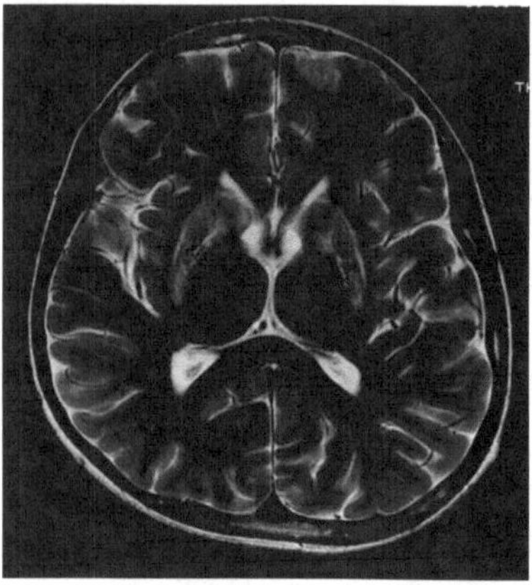

Figure 6.12: Axial T2-weighted MR image showing hyperintensities in bilateral putamen and caudate nucleus in a case of Wilson's disease

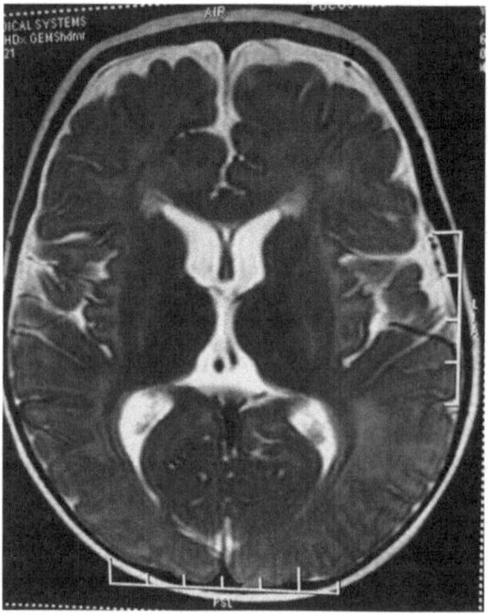

Figure 6.13: Axial T2-weighted MR image showing demyelination involving periventricular and parieto-occipital white matter in a case of Krabbe disease

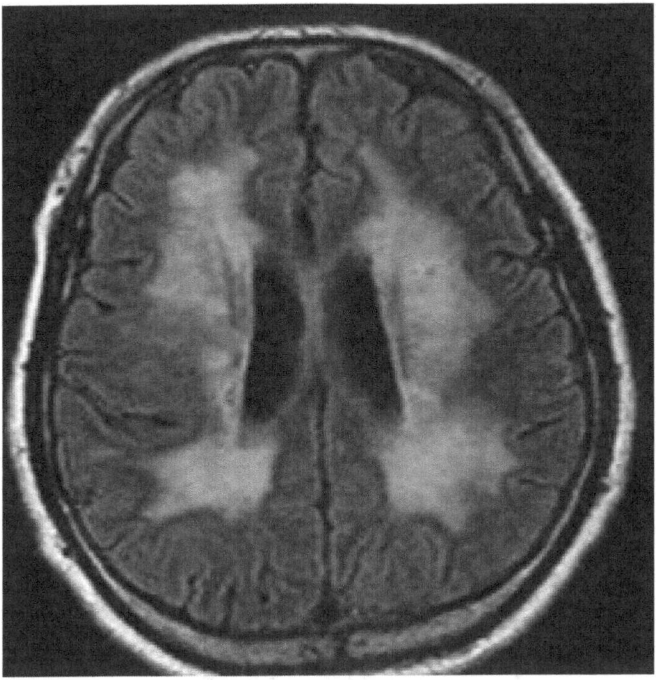

Figure 6.14: Axial FLAIR MR image showing near complete lack of myelination in a case of metachromatic leukodystrophy

INTRACRANIAL HAEMORRHAGE

Extradural Hemorrhage (EDH)	Subdural Hemorrhage (SDH)
Due to laceration of meningeal artery or dural sinus	Tearing of bridging cortical veins
Fracture common, biconvex, does not cross sutures	Fracture uncommon, crescentric, cross sutures

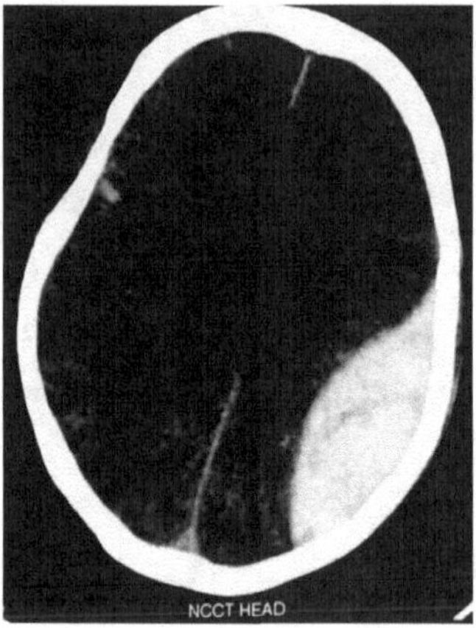

Figure 6.15: Axial non-contrast CT head showing biconvex shaped extra-axial hyperdense collection in left parieto-occipital region and along falx cerebri suggestive of extradural haemorrhage. Also note is made of small contusion in right parietal region

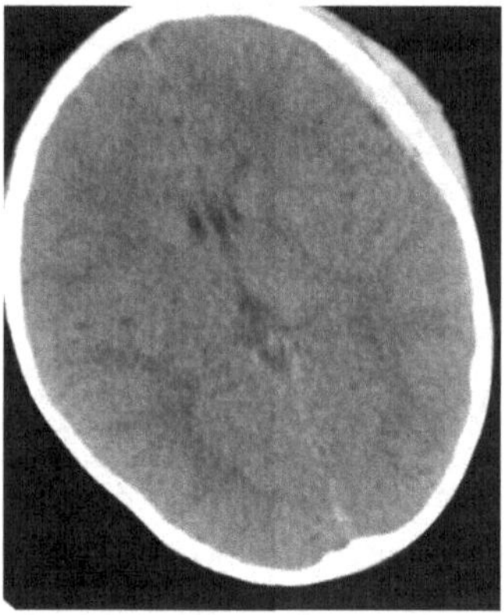

Figure 6.16: Axial non-contrast CT head showing crescent shaped extra-axial hyperdense collection in left frontal region suggestive of subdural haemorrhage associated with scalp hematoma

HYDROCEPHALUS

Obstructive Hydrocephalus	**Non-Obstructive Hydrocephalus**
Passage of CSF within the ventricular system or in the subarachnoid space is impaired at some point. **Communicating obstructive hydrocephalus** • Often merely referred to as communicating hydrocephalus • Passage of CSF from the ventricular system and into the subarachnoid space is unimpeded but absorption of CFS via arachnoid granulations is impaired • Most commonly seen as a result of subarachnoid hemorrhage or meningitis • Extra-axial CSF spaces are also distended • Seen as a result of subarachnoid hemorrhage, meningitis **Non-communicating obstructive hydrocephalus** • Often merely referred to as obstructive hydrocephalus • Due to obstruction of CSF outflow at any point (e.g. aqueduct stenosis, foramen of Monro, trapped fourth ventricle, ependymitis) • Up-stream ventricles are dilated and exert mass effect upon adjacent brain	Often referred to as ex-vacuo dilatation of the ventricles • Up-stream ventricles are dilated and exert mass effect upon adjacent brain • CSF can pass out of the ventricles and into the basal cisterns without impediment, and is readily absorbed • Ventricles are enlarged due to loss of adjacent brain parenchyma **Benign communicating hydrocephalus/benign external hydrocephalus/benign enlargement of subarachnoid space** • Due to chronic subdural hygroma of infancy • Enlargement of subarachnoid spaces greater than 5 mm (frontal and temporal regions)

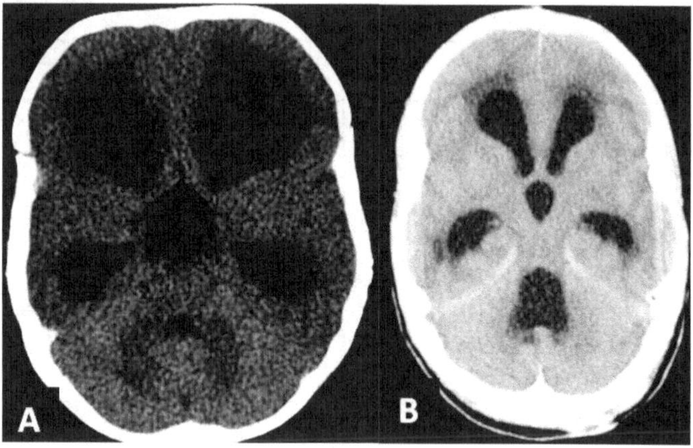

Figure 6.17: (A) Axial non-contrast CT head showing dilated frontal, temporal horns; dilated third ventricle and collapsed fourth ventricle suggestive of non-communicating obstructive hydrocephalus in case of aqueductal stenosis (B) Axial non-contrast CT head showing dilated supratentorial and infratentorial ventricles suggestive of communicating obstructive hydrocephalus in a case of subarachnoid hemorrhage

TUBEROUS SCLEROSIS

Clinical triad of popular facial lesions, seizures, mental retardation.

Imaging Findings:

CNS Lesions

Cortical tubers – T1 hyper/T2 hypointense lesions in neonates and young children; T2 hyperintense in older children.

Benign white matter lesions – Seen on T2 weighed MR image as any one of the four types: straight or curvilinear bands extending from ventricles towards the cortex, wedge-shaped lesions, cerebellar lesions or tumefactive lesions.

Subependymal nodules – Located near the caudate nucleus near the striothalamic groove.

Subependymal giant cell astrocytoma – Located at foramen of Monro.

Kidneys – Cysts, angiomyolipomas.

CVS – Cardiac rhabdomyoma, aneurysms, stenosis.

Liver – Leiomyoma, adenomas.

Spleen and pancreatic adenomas.

Musculoskeletal – Bony islands, cysts, periosteal new bone.

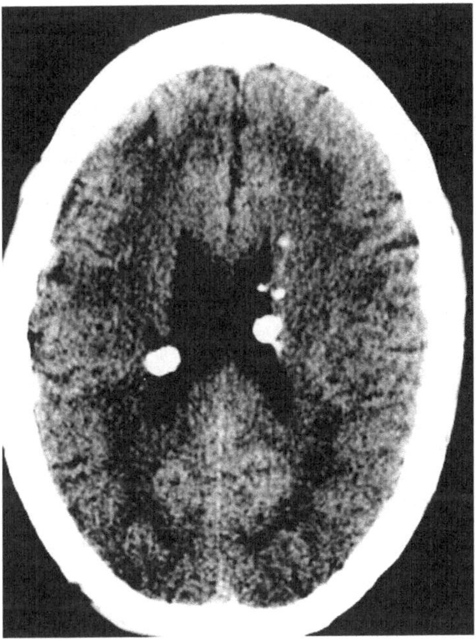

Figure 6.18: Axial non-contrast CT head showing calcified subependymal nodules in a case of tuberous sclerosis

HYPOXIC–ISCHAEMIC ENCEPHALOPATHY (HIE)

MRI is the most sensitive and specific imaging technique.

Sonography is sensitive for the detection of haemorrhage, periventricular leukomalacia (PVL) and hydrocephalus.

Preterm Neonate: Injury to Periventricular White Matter

Term Infant: Subcortical White Matter and Para Sagittal Cortical Injury

Initial ultrasound shows echogenic changes in periventricular/subcortical regions, cysts formation, cystic encephalomalacia, thin and gracile corpus callosum, peritrigonal hyperintensities, undulating ventricular borders.

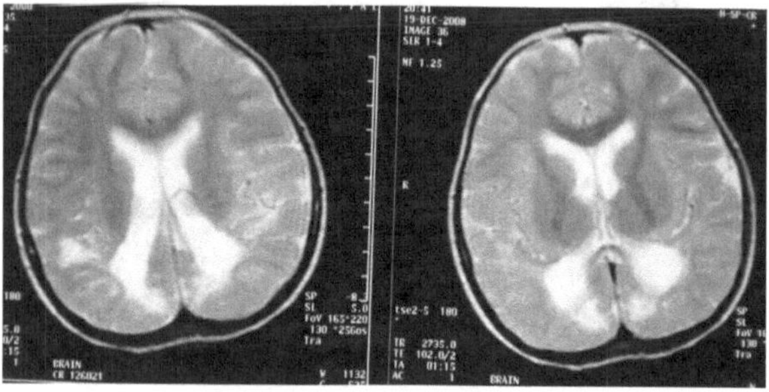

Figure 6.19: Axial T2-weighted MR brain scan showing peritrigonal hyperintensities with undulating occipital horns in a case of HIE

BRAIN ABSCESS

Four stages are recognized, which distinct pathological and radiological features:

1. Early cerebritis.
2. Late cerebritis.
3. Early capsule.
4. Late capsule.

Risk factors: Congenital heart disease, bacterial endocarditis, intravenous drug abuse, lung infections, dental abscess, systemic sepsis.

CT:

Iso to hyperdense ring with central low attenuation, surrounding vasogenic edema, ventriculitis.

MRI:

MRI is more sensitive and especially with the addition MRS and DWI far more specific for the diagnosis of cerebral abscesses.

T1: Central low intensity.

T2/FLAIR: Central high signal intensity with peripheral edema.

DWI/ADC: Diffusion restriction.

T1 post contrast: Thick irregular enhancing rim.

MR spectroscopy - Elevation of a succinate peak is relatively specific but not present in all abscesses; high lactate, acetate, alanine, valine, leucine and isoleucine levels peak may be present; Cho/Crn and NAA peaks are reduced.

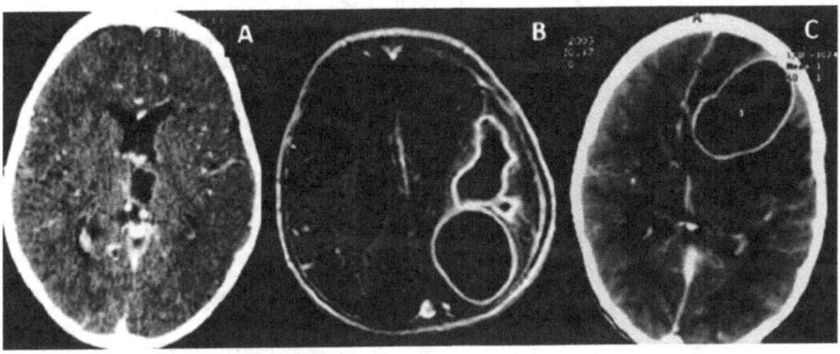

Figure 6.20: Axial contrast CT head showing brain abscesses in three different cases

CNS TUBERCULOSIS

Tubercular Meningitis

1. Leptomeningitis–Characterized by thick tuberculous exudates in subarachnoid spaces.
2. Pachymeningitis–Characterized by plaque like leptomeningeal thickening.

Tuberculoma

Focal tuberculous cerebritis: Seen as focal gyral enhancement.

Tuberculous encephalopathy: Seen as severe unilateral or bilateral cerebral edema.

AIDS related tuberculosis: Infarction, meningeal enhancement and parenchymal disease are more florid in HIV related tuberculosis.

Complications:

1. Cerebral infarction secondary to obliterative end arteritis.
2. Hydrocephalus due to arachnoid fibrosis.

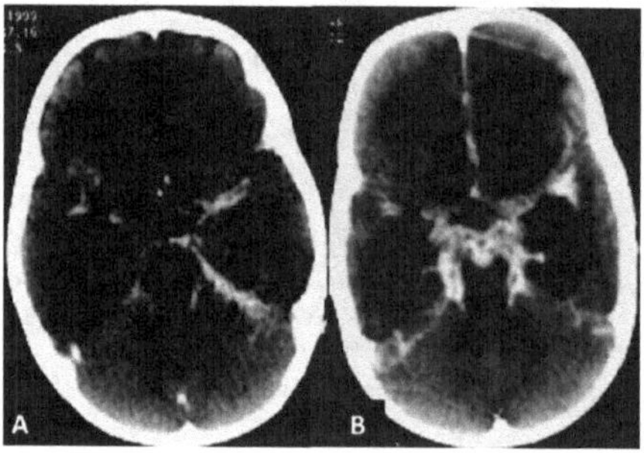

Figure 6.21: (A) CECT head showing enhancing meninges along tentorium and exudates in a case of pyogenic meningitis (B) CECT head showing basal exudates with moderate hydrocephalus in a case of tubercular meningitis

VIRAL ENCEPHALITIS

1. *Herpes Simplex:* MRI shows hyperintensities in bilateral medial temporal lobes, insular region and cingulate gyrus with sparing of putamen. Haemorrhage is suggestive of fulminant encephalitis. Patchy contrast enhancement may be seen.
2. *Creutzfeldt-Jakob disease:* High T2 signal in putamen, posterior thalami and caudate head (these changes are better appreciated on FLAIR).
3. *Subacute sclerosing panencephalitis:* Occurs after measles infection. MRI reveals gross atrophy and non-specific T2 and FLAIR hyperintensities in cerebral and cerebellar white matter.
4. *Rasmussen's encephalitis:* MRI shows unilateral cortical atrophy and non-specific unilateral brain changes.
5. *Polio:* Increased T2W signal in spinal cord and brainstem involvement.
6. *HIV encephalitis:* Cerebral atrophy, T2W hyperintensities in white matter and basal ganglia.
7. *Japanese encephalitis:* T2 hyperintensities in basal ganglia and thalamus.

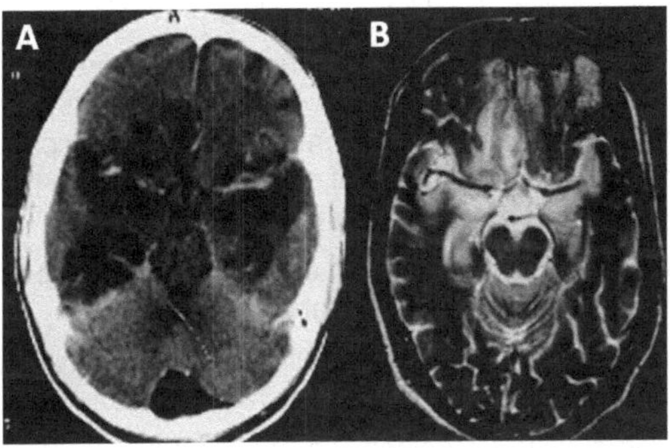

Figure 6.22: (A) Axial CT head showing hypodensities in bilateral temporal lobes (B) Axial T2-weighted MR brain image showing hyperintensities in bilateral medial temporal lobes, insular region and cingulate gyrus in a case of herpes simplex encephalitis

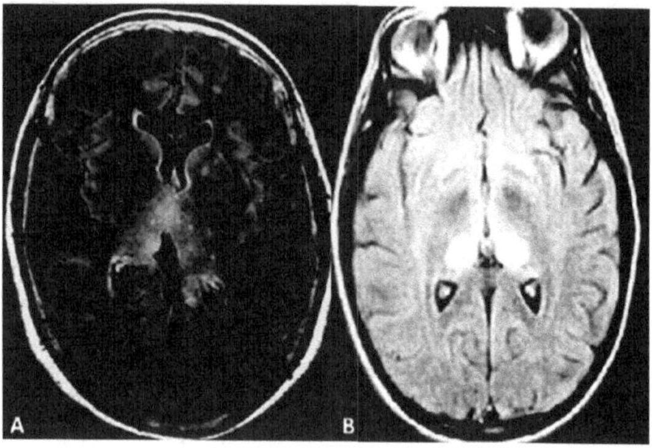

Figure 6.23: (A) Axial T2-weighted MR brain image showing hyperintensities in bilateral thalami in a case of Japanese encephalitis (B) Axial T2-weighted MR FLAIR image showing hyperintense T2 signal in bilateral posterior thalami in a case of Creutzfeldt-Jakob disease

HIV INVOLVEMENT IN BRAIN

1. *HIV Encephalitis* – Cerebral atrophy, T2W hyperintensities in white matter and basal ganglia.
2. *Progressive multifocal leukoencephalopathy* – It is caused by JC virus. MR brain reveals extensive asymmetric T2 hyperintensities in periventricular and subcortical white matter with involvement of subcortical U-fibres. No cerebral atrophy and mass effect is seen.
3. *Cryptococcus* – Features of meningitis; punctuate foci of increased T2 signal in basal ganglia and pons.
4. *Toxoplasma* – Solitary or multiple ring enhancing lesions in basal ganglia, thalami and grey-white matter junction.
5. *Tuberculosis* – Meningitis; tuberculomas.
6. *Lymphoma* – Periventricular T2 hyperintensities without mass effect with subependymal spread.

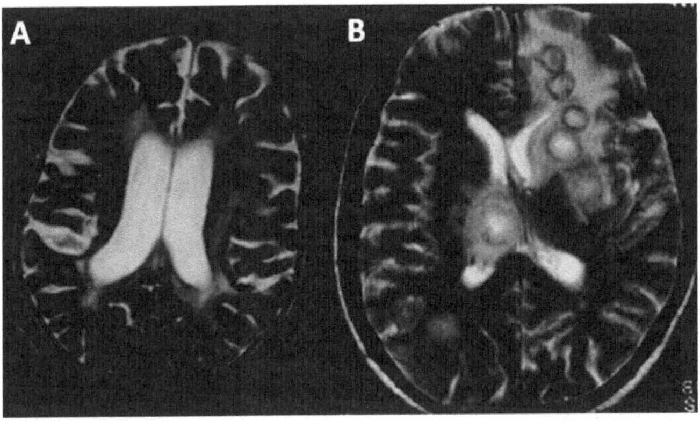

Figure 6.24: (A) Axial T2-weighted MR brain image showing symmetrical periventricular demyelination in a case of HIV encephalitis (B) Axial T2-weighted MR brain image showing target like lesions in a case of toxoplasmosis

CONGENITAL CNS INFECTIONS

1. *Cytomegalovirus:* Calcification in periventricular region (germinal matrix region), microcephaly, polymicrogyria.
2. *Toxoplasma:* Calcification in cerebral cortex, basal ganglia more common; calcification less common in periventricular location.
3. *HIV:* Diffuse cerebral atrophy; basal ganglia calcification in first year of life.
4. *Herpes simplex:* Meningitis; limbic system involvement; atrophy.
5. *Rubella:* Microcephaly, atrophy, chorioretinitis and parenchymal calcifications.

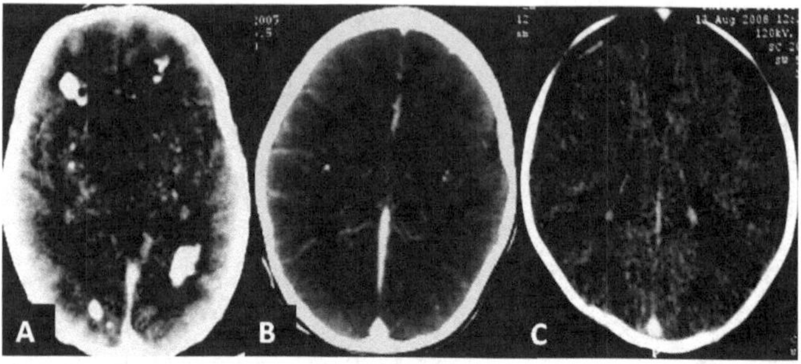

Figure 6.25: Axial CT head scan showing (A) periventricular calcifications in a case of congenital CMV infection (B) calcification in cerebral cortex in a case of toxoplasma (C) cerebral atrophy in a case of congenital HIV infection

DISORDERS OF NEURONAL MIGRATION

1. *Lissencephaly:* Agyria-pachygyria complex with poorly formed gyri and sulci giving a figure of 8 appearance due to shallow vertical sylvian fissure.
2. *Schizencephaly:* Clefts extending through the full-thickness of the cerebral mantle from ventricle to cortical surface lined by heterotopic grey matter.
3. *Heterotopic grey matter:* Collection of abnormal grey matter in subependymal region or in white matter.
4. *Cortical dysplasia:* Focal disorganization of cerebral cortex appearing as expanded gyrus.

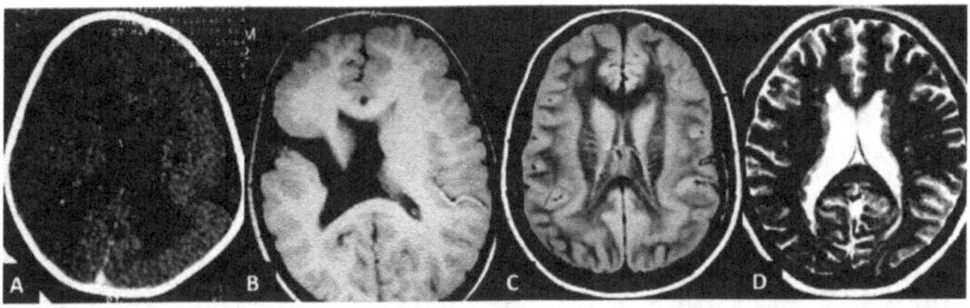

Figure 6.26: Axial CT head showing (A) Lissencephaly (B) MR FLAIR image showing schizencephaly (C) Axial MR FLAIR image showing band heterotopia (D) Axial T2-weighted MR brain image showing subependymal heterotopia

ULTRASOUND CRANIUM

Grading of Intracranial Haemorrhage

Grade I – Haemorrhage limited to subependymal region.

Grade II – Haemorrhage extending into ventricular system without ventriculomegaly.

Grade III – Haemorrhage extending into ventricular system with ventriculomegaly.

Grade IV – Any grade with haemorrhage extending into the brain tissue.

Periventricular Leukomalacia (PVL)

PVL is also known as Hypoxic-Ischemic Encephalopathy (HIE) of the preterm. It is a white matter disease that affects the periventricular zones. In preterm neonates, this white matter zone is a watershed zone between deep and superficial vessels. PVL presents as areas of increased periventricular echogenicity. Normally the echogenicity of the periventricular white matter should be less than the echogenicity of the choroid plexus.

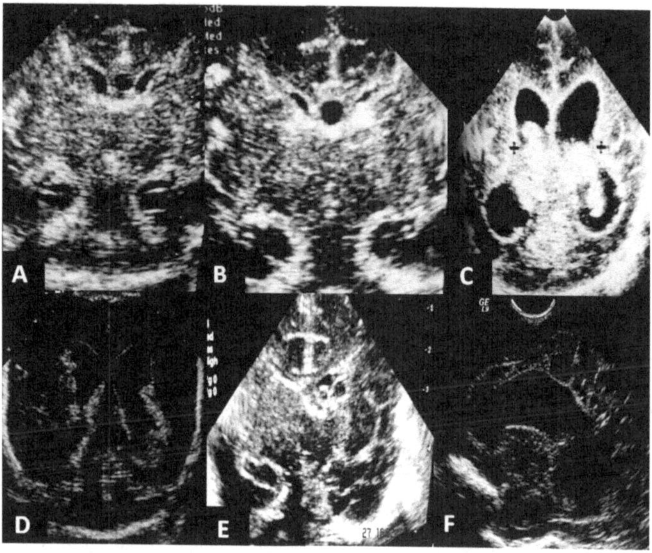

Figure 6.27: Ultrasound cranium showing (A) Normal cranial ultrasound (B) Grade II intracranial hemorrhage (C) Grade III intracranial hemorrhage (D) Grade IV intracranial hemorrhage (E,F) Periventricular leukomalacia with subependymal and periventricular cysts

CNS TUMORS

Supratentorial	Infratentorial
Intraparenchymal	Astrocytoma
Astrocytoma	Medulloblastoma
Ependymoma	Ependymoma
Dysembryoblastic neuroepithelial tumor (DNET)	Brainstem glioma
	Dermoid/Epidermoid
Ganglioglioma/Gangliocytoma	

Contd.

Contd.

Teratoma Primitive neuroectodermal tumor (PNET) Atypical teratoid/rhabdoid tumor ***Extra-axial*** Choroid plexus papilloma/ carcinoma Langerhans cell histiocytosis Epidermoid/Dermoid Arachnoid cyst Metastasis ***Sellar/Suprasellar*** Craniopharyngioma Astrocytoma Rathke cleft cyst Germ cell tumors Hypothalamic hamartoma Langerhans cell histiocytosis Pituitary adenoma	Schwannoma/meningioma

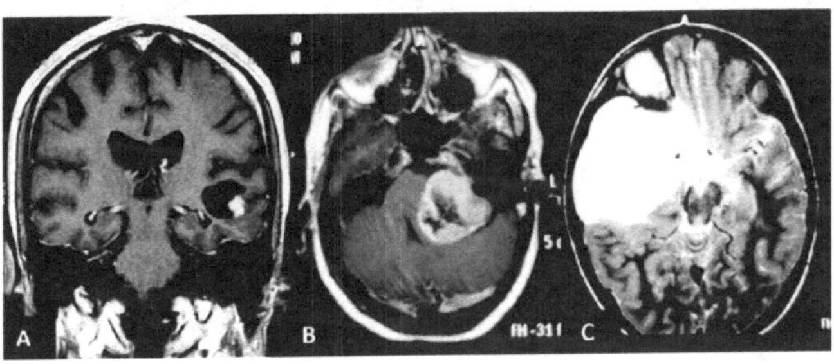

Figure 6.28: (A) Coronal MR image showing left temporal lobe pilocystic astrocytoma (B) Axial contrast MR image showing left acoustic schwannoma (C) T2-weighted axial MR image showing arachnoid cyst

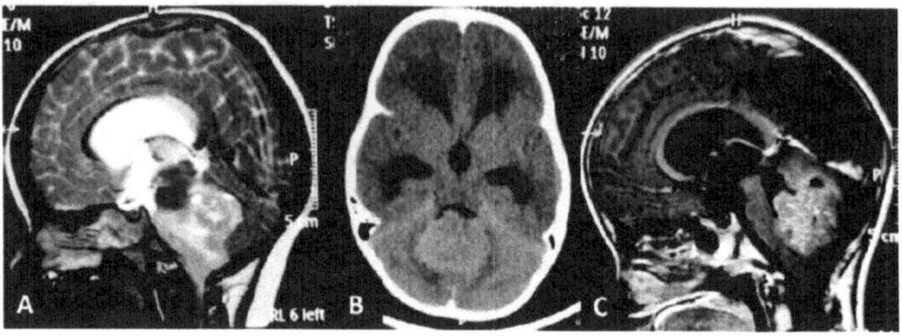

Figure 6.29: (A) Sagittal T2-weighted MR image showing heterogenous hyperintense lesion in the region of fourth ventricle extending into spinal canal suggestive of Ependymoma (B) Axial NCCT head showing hyperdense lesion in infratentorial location causing upstream hydrocephalus in a case of medulloblastoma (C) Same case sagittal T1 contrast MR image showing heterogenously enhancing lesion in 4th ventricle

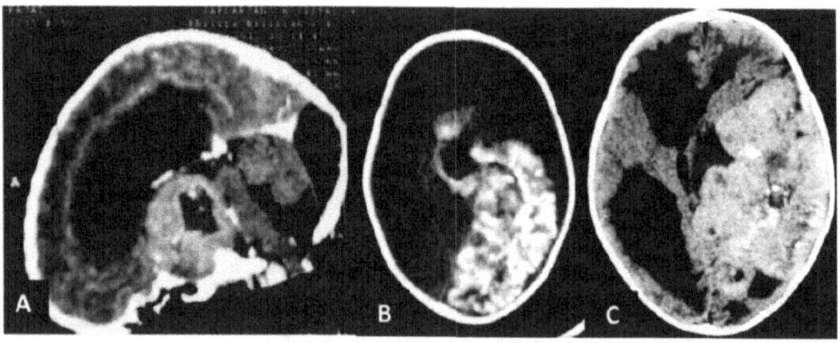

Figure 6.30: (A) Sagittal contrast CT image showing heterogenously enhancing lesion in sella-suprasellar location with calcification in case of craniopharyngioma (B) Axial contrast CT head showing choroid plexus carcinoma (C) Axial contrast CT head showing primitive neuroectodermal tumor (PNET)

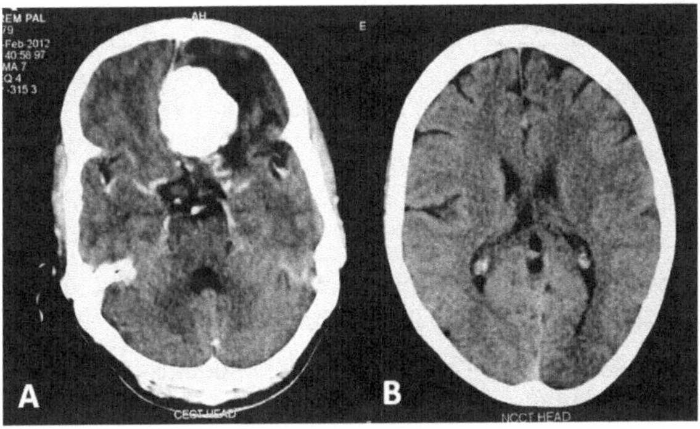

Figure 6.31: (A) Axial contrast CT head showing left parafalcine meningioma with surrounding edema (B) Axial NCCT head showing corpus callosum lipoma

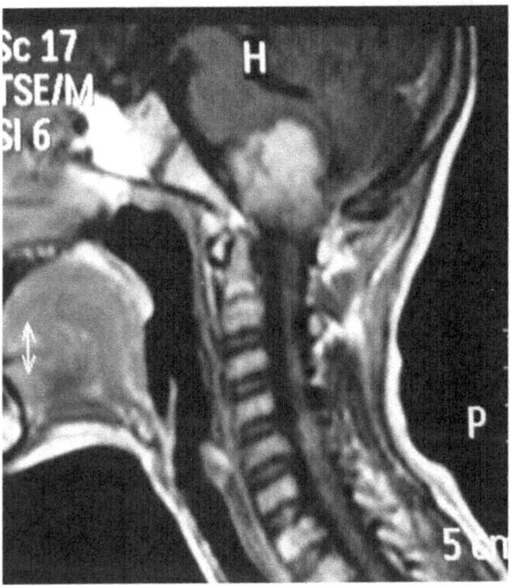

Figure 6.32: T1 contrast sagittal MR image showing brainstem astrocytoma

MULTIPLE SCLEROSIS AND ADEM

Multiple Sclerosis:

Relapsing and remitting illness.

Demyelinating disease where there is dissemination in space, time. It is a clinical diagnosis.

MRI: Periventricular white matter hyperintensity, right angled to ventricular surface, ovoid >3 mm, Dawson's finger.

Corpus callosum is typically involved especially the calloso-septal interface.

Acute and subacute stage, lesions may show enhancement.

Cerebral atrophy seen in late stages.

Spinal cord involvement: Cervical and thoracic cord more often involved - focal T2 hyperintense lesions which are seen in eccentric in peripheral dorsolateral aspect of cordless than 2 vertebral segments of cord involvement is usually seen.

Spinal cord atrophy may be seen in chronic stage and in acute and subacute stage, spinal cord expansion and edema is seen.

ADEM

Usually Monophasic Illness

Widespread autoimmune CNS inflammation triggered by infection/vaccination.

Post-infective – Measles, chickenpox, rubella, URTI.

Post vaccination – Rabies, yellow fever, influenza.

MRI: Usually asymmetric, bilateral T2 hyperintense lesions in white matter of cerebrum, cerebellum, brainstem, spinal cord. Grey matter especially that of basal ganglia is also often involved. Involvement of callososeptal interface is unusual.

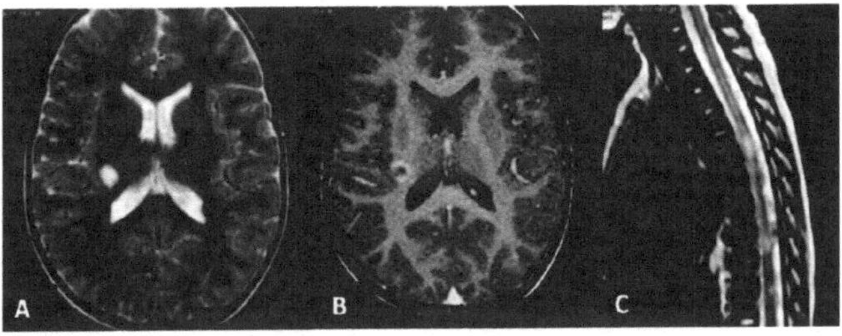

Figure 6.33: Case of multiple sclerosis showing (A) T2-weighted axial MR brain image showing focal hyperintense lesion in right periventricular white matter (B) Axial contrast MR image showing incomplete ring enhancement (C) T2-sagittal MR image of dorsal spine showing hyperintense plaques

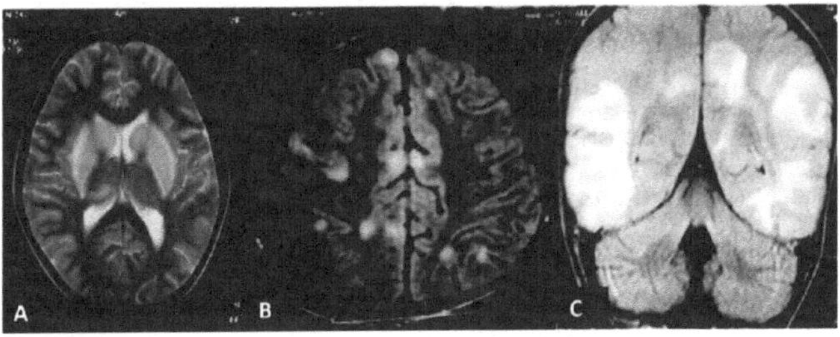

Figure 6.34: Three cases of ADEM in three different patients (A) T2-weighted MR brain image showing hyperintensities in bilateral basal ganglia and right thalamus (B) Axial FLAIR brain image showing focal discrete hyperintensities in subcortical white matter (C) Coronal FLAIR image showing large tumefactive lesions in bilateral white matter

7

Chapter

Genitourinary System

INTRAVENOUS UROGRAPHY

Immediate Faint Persistent Nephrogram

1. Acute glomerulonephritis.
2. Renal vein thrombosis.
3. Chronic ischemia.

Immediate Distinct Persistent Nephrogram

1. Acute tubular necrosis.
2. Acute renal failure.
3. Acute hypotension.

Increasingly Dense Nephrogram

1. Acute obstruction.
2. Acute hypotension.
3. Acute tubular necrosis.
4. Acute pyelonephritis.
5. Multiple myeloma.
6. Renal vein thrombosis.
7. Acute glomerulonephritis.
8. Acute papillary necrosis.
9. Amyloid.

Striated Nephrogram

1. Acute ureteric obstruction.
2. Infantile polycystic disease.

3. Medullary sponge kidney.
4. Acute pyelonephritis.

Rim Nephrogram

1. Severe hydronephrosis.
2. Acute arterial obstruction.

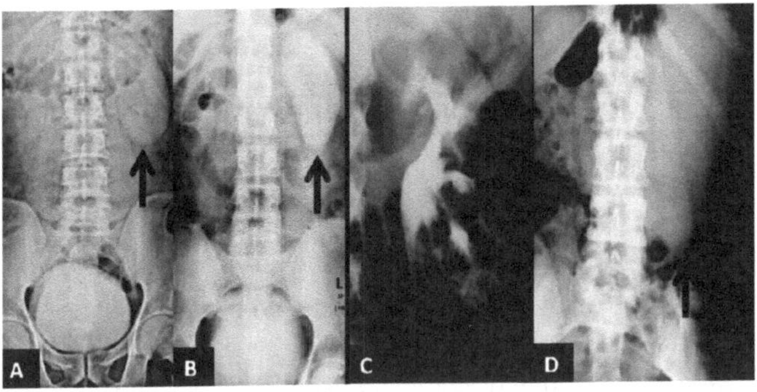

Figure 7.1: IVU films showing (A) persistent nephrogram (B) increasingly dense nephrogram (C) striated nephrogram (D) rim nephrogram

GRADING OF HYDRONEPHROSIS

Grade I (mild) - Dilatation of the renal pelvis without dilatation of the calyces (can also occur in the extra-renal pelvis); no parenchymal atrophy.

Grade II (mild) - Dilatation of the renal pelvis (mild) and calyces (pelvicalyceal pattern is retained); no parenchymal atrophy.

Grade III (moderate) - Dilatation of the renal pelvis and calyces; blunting of forncies and flattening of papillae; mild cortical thinning may be seen.

Grade IV (severe/gross) - Gross dilatation of the renal pelvis and calyces, which appear ballooned; loss of borders between the renal pelvis and calyces; renal atrophy seen as cortical thinning.

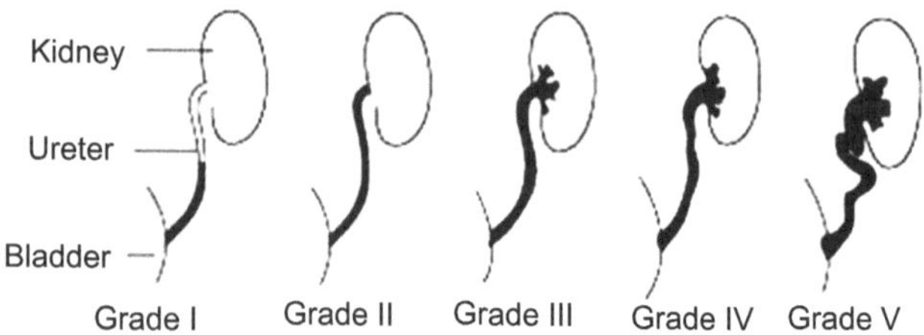

Figure 7.2: Figure showing grading of hydronephrosis

GRADING OF VESICOURETERIC REFLUX

Grade I - Reflux limited to ureter.

Grade II - Reflux into renal pelvis.

Grade III - Mild dilatation of ureter and pelvicalyceal system

Grade IV - Tortuous ureter with moderate dilatation; blunting of fornices but preserved papillary impressions

Grade V - Tortuous ureter with severe dilatation of ureter and pelvicalyceal system; loss of fornicies and papillary impressions

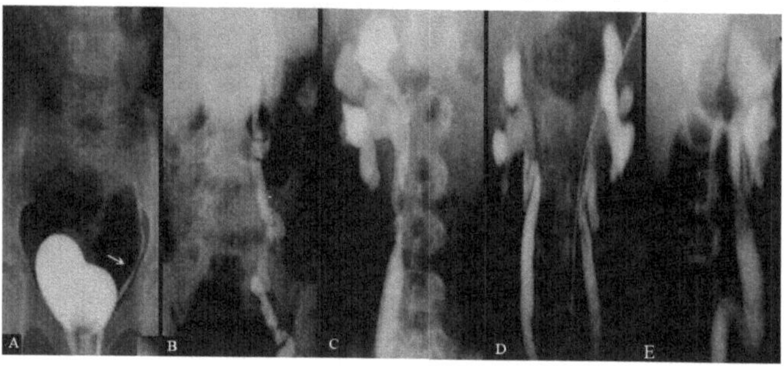

Figure 7.3: Voiding cystourethrography (VCUG) images show International Grading System of vesicoureteral reflux (VUR)—(A) grade I, (B) grade II (C) grade III (D) grade IV and (E) grade V. In grade I (A), contrast material reaches distal ureter (arrow). Contrast reaches renal pelvis in grades II to V, with increasingly severe pelvicalyceal and ureteral dilatation

POSTERIOR URETHRAL VALVE

Ultrasound

The bladder is typically thick-walled and trabeculated with an elongated and dilated posterior urethra (keyhole sign). The kidneys in most cases are hydronephrotic.

Examination of the posterior urethra can be performed longitudinally through the perineum. Ideally this is performed during micturition (which may take some patience) at which time the proximal urethra can be seen to dilate. A diameter of more than 6 mm is considered abnormal and is highly specific and sensitive to the diagnosis. Additionally the valve may actually be seen as an echogenic line.

Voiding Cystourethrogram (VCUG)

It is the best imaging technique for the diagnosis of posterior urethral valves. The diagnosis is best made during the micturition phase in lateral or oblique views, such that the posterior urethra can be imaged adequately.

On VCUG: Dilatation and elongation of the posterior urethra, linear radiolucent band corresponding to the valve (only occasionally seen), VUR, bladder trabeculations or diverticulae may be seen.

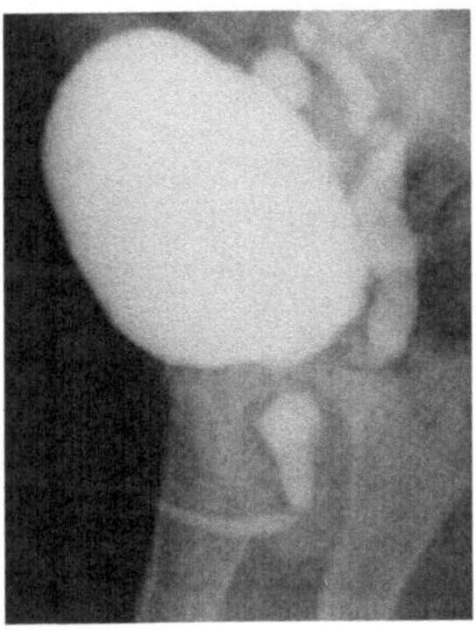

Figure 7.4: VCUG study showing posterior urethral valve with VUR and hutch diverticulum in bladder

HORSESHOE KIDNEY

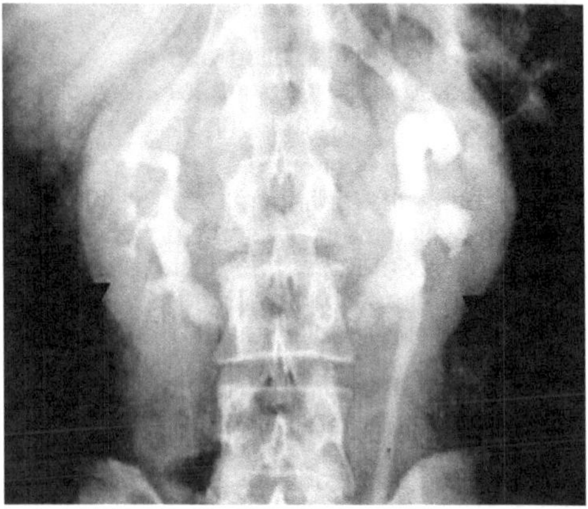

Figure 7.5: IVP film showing classical case of horseshoe kidney with fusion of isthmus across the midline

Associations

Horseshoe kidneys are frequently associated with both genitourinary and non-genitourinary malformations. Various syndromes associated are:

Down's syndrome, Turner syndrome, Edward syndrome, Patau syndrome, Ellis-van-Crevald syndrome, Fanconi anemia, Glotz syndrome, Kabuki syndrome, Pallister-Hall syndrome, VACTERL association.

Complications: Hydronephrosis, PUJO, infection, renal calculi, increased incidence of malignancy – Wilms tumour, transitional cell carcinoma (TCC), increased susceptibility to trauma.

Imaging Features

On imaging, horseshoe kidneys may be identified on abdominal radiographs. Four kinds of abnormal renal outlines suggestive of horseshoe kidney are: lower than normal, too close to the spine, vertical long axis and visible isthmus.

On excretory urography, 'hand-holding calyces' and 'flower-vase' appearance is seen.

CT and MRI

May be done for confirmation. Both CT and MRI demonstrate normal renal parenchyma, but with abnormal configuration. Enhancement is normal, and excretory phase imaging may be used to assess the collecting system.

URETEROCELE

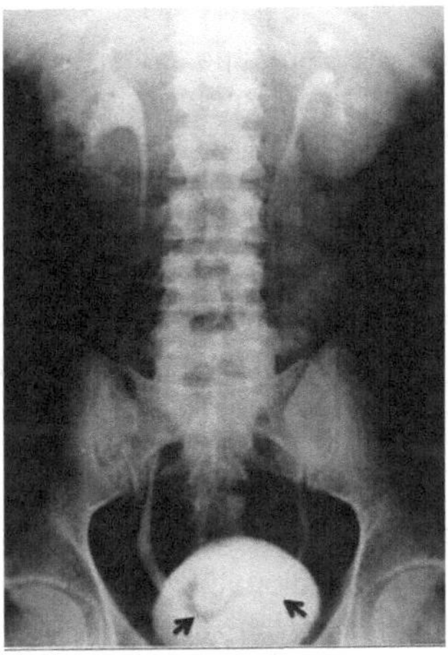

Figure 7.6: Intravenous urography film demonstrating bilateral ureterocele (arrow) larger in size on the right side

Ureterocele is ballooning of the distal end of the ureter. Ureteroceles may be associated with either a single or a duplex ureter.

Types:

(a) Simple/intravesical ureterocele–Orifice of the ureter and the ureterocele are intravesical.

(b) Ectopic ureterocele – Ureterocele lies in the submucosa of the bladder and may extend into the bladder neck/urethra.

On US, simple ureterocele is seen as a cystic intravesical mass. With real-time US, partial or complete collapse of a simple ureterocele secondary to ureteric peristalsis can be demonstrated. At VCUG, a collapsed simple ureterocele usually manifests as a rounded filling defect within the bladder. IVU shows the classic "cobra head" appearance consisting of a round or oval area of increased opacity surrounded by the radiolucent halo.

Pseudoureteroceles are rare and consist of two types – (i) coiled uniformly dilated distal segment of the ureter forming a submucosal mass (ii) ectopic ureter draining into a mesonephric duct cyst.

MEGAURETER

Megaureter is defined as presence of an enlarged ureter (>7 mm) with or without concomitant dilatation of the upper collecting system.

Types

(a) **Primary** - Primary megaureter includes all cases of megaureter due to an idiopathic congenital alteration at the vesicoureteral junction. There are three subtypes: obstructed primary megaureter refluxing primary megaureter and nonrefluxing unobstructed primary megaureter.

In obstructed primary megaureter, there is dilatation above a short (0.5–4 cm), aperistaltic, normal-caliber juxtavesical section of a normally inserted ureter. Refluxing primary megaureter is caused by a short or absent intravesical ureter, congenital paraureteric diverticulum, or other derangement of the vesicoureteral junction.

(b) **Secondary -** Secondary megaureter occurs as a result of some abnormality involving the bladder or urethra.

On imaging, first voiding cystourethrography is performed to exclude vesicoureteral reflux. US reveals hydronephrosis and ureteral dilatation above the persistently narrowed distal aperistaltic segment.

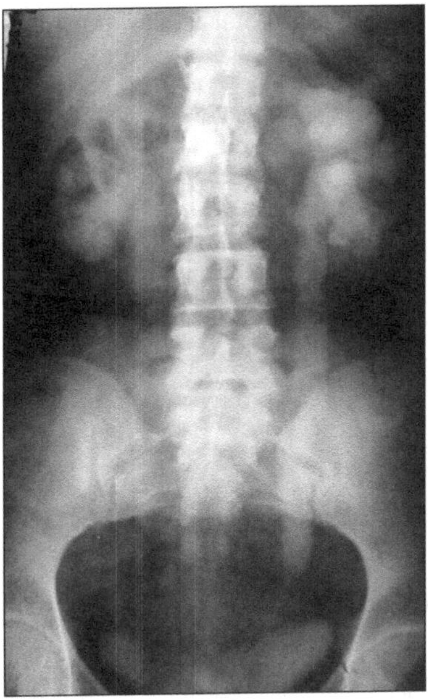

Figure 7.7: IVU film showing bilateral megaureter with hydronephrosis

RETROCAVAL URETER

Retrocaval or circumcaval ureter results from anomalous development of the infra-renal portion of inferior vena cava (IVC) and not from anomalous development of the ureter. There is anomalous development of the infrarenal IVC from the right posterior cardinal vein that is embryologically more medial. Classically, the ureter crosses posterior to the IVC and then travel medially and anteriorly to partially circumscribe the IVC.

Types: Type 1- Moderate hydronephrosis with deviation of the ureteral segment medial to the pedicle of L3 vertebral level resulting in "S" or "fish hook" deformity. Type 2 - There is mild hydronephrosis and the ureter is sickle shaped at the level of obstruction.

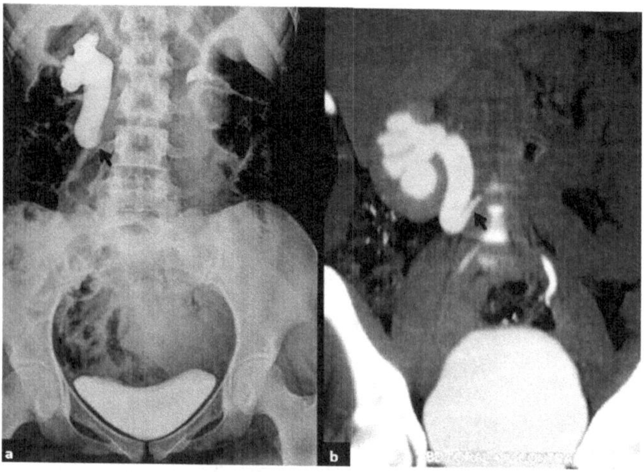

Figure 7.8: (a) Intravenous urography film showing reverse-J shape of upper right ureter (arrow) and moderate proximal hydroureteronephrosis suggestive of retrocaval ureter (b) Coronal contrast-enhanced MIP images confirming the same findings (arrow)

On imaging, IVU shows characteristic reverse - J appearance due to medial deviation of the ureters with moderate proximal hydroureteronephrosis.

PELVI-URETERIC JUNCTION OBSTRUCTION (PUJO)

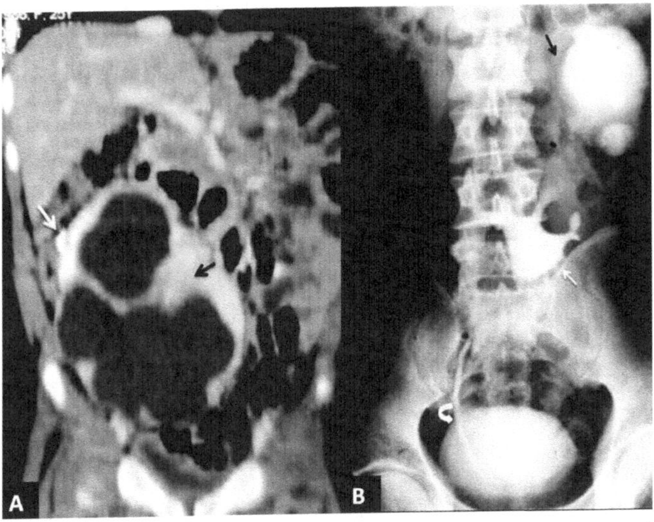

Figure 7.9: (A) Coronal contrast-enhanced CT scan in same case of ureteropelvic junction obstruction (PUJO) of right crossed fused ectopic kidney showing excretion of contrast in displaced pelvicalyceal system (white arrow) and PUJO (black arrow) of crossed fused ectopic kidney. (B) Intravenous urography film in a case of left crossed fused ectopia showing ureteropelvic junction obstruction (black arrow) of the orthotopic kidney and crossed fused ectopic kidney (white arrow) located caudally and its ureter (curved arrow) crossing and opening in its normal position

It is one of the causes of an obstructive uropathy. It can be congenital or acquired with a congenital PUJ obstruction being one of the most common causes of antenatal hydronephrosis.

Imaging Features

IVU

Traditionally intravenous urogram (IVU) has been performed for assessing for PUJ obstruction. The administration of furosemide is used to assist confirming the diagnosis, in particular to identify complete or partial PUJO and to differentiate between non-obstructed extrarenal pelvis.

Ultrasound: Shows evidence of disproportionately dilated renal pelvis with a collapsed proximal ureter.

CT: May show evidence of hydronephrosis with or without calyectasis and non-dilated ureters. May also show crossing vessels at the PUJ especially when surgical intervention is planned.

Scintigraphy: ^{99m}Tc diethylenetriaminepentaacetic acid (DTPA) or ^{99m}Tc MAG3 (agent of choice).

NEUROGENIC BLADDER

Classification

1. *Sensory neurogenic bladder* - Posterior columns of the spinal cord or afferent tracts leading from the bladder.
2. *Motor paralytic bladder* - Damage to motor neurons of the bladder.
3. *Uninhibited neurogenic bladder* - Incomplete spinal cord lesions above S2 or cerebral cortex or cerebropontine axis lesions.
4. *Reflex neurogenic bladder* - Complete spinal cord lesions above S2 - may lead to cone bladder.
5. *Autonomous neurogenic bladder* - Conus or cauda equina lesions.

Imaging Features

Generally a markedly contracted or distended bladder, with trabeculated thick-walled bladder resembling 'Christmas tree'.

Significant post void residual urine is also noted.

Often associated with spinal, sacral anomalies and renal anomalies.

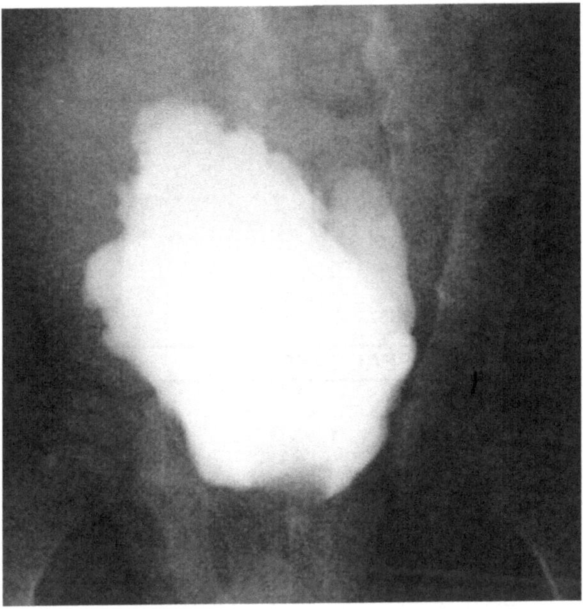

Figure 7.10: VCUG film showing irregular trabeculated neurogenic bladder with vesicoureteric reflux

8

Chapter

Miscellaneous

LUCENT METAPHYSEAL BAND

1. Normal neonates.
2. Metaphyseal fracture.
3. Healing rickets.
4. Leukaemia.
5. Lymphoma.
6. Metastatic neuroblastoma.
7. Congenital infections.
8. Scurvy.
9. Any severe illness.

DENSE METAPHYSEAL BAND

1. Normal neonate.
2. Lead poisoning.
3. Congenital hypothyroidism.
4. Osteopetrosis.
5. Hypervitaminosis D.
6. Radiation.

ALTERNATE RADIOLUCENT AND DENSE METAPHYSEAL BANDS

1. Rickets especially Vitamin D-dependent rickets.
2. Osteopetrosis.
3. Chronic anaemias.
4. Treated leukaemia, lymphoma.
5. Post chemotherapy.
6. Growth arrest lines.

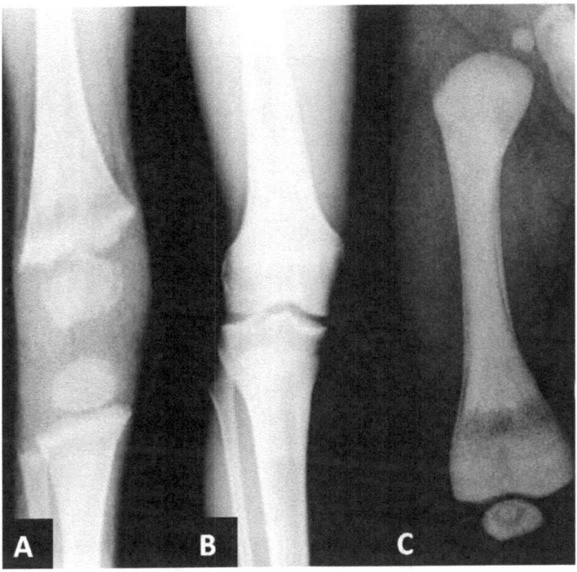

Figure 8.1: Radiographs showing (A) lucent metaphyseal band (B) dense metaphyseal band and (C) alternate dense and lucent metaphyseal bands

FRAYING OF METAPHYSES

1. Rickets.
2. Hypophosphatasia.
3. Copper deficiency.
4. Chronic stress.

RETARDED SKELETAL MATURATION

1. Congenital heart disease.
2. Malnutrition.
3. Rickets.

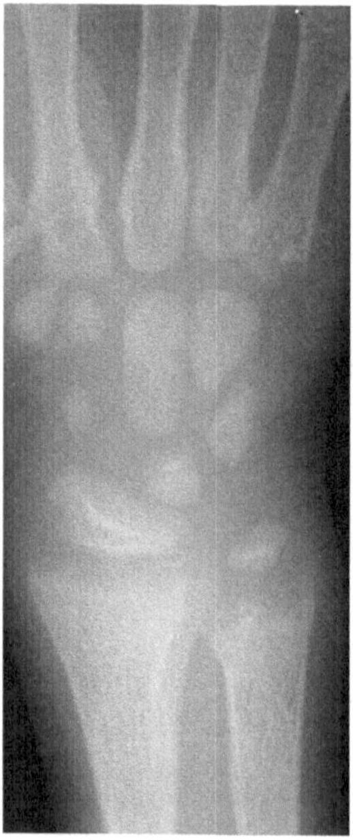

Figure 8.2: Radiograph showing metaphyseal fraying in a case of rickets

4. Maternal deprivation.
5. Hypothyroidism.
6. Hypopituitarism.
7. Trisomy 21.
8. Renal failure.
9. Inflammatory bowel disease.
10. Congenital syndromes.

GENERALIZED ACCELERATED SKELETAL MATURATION

1. Idiopathic sexual precocity.
2. Adrenal and gonadal tumors.
3. Hyperthyroidism.
4. McCune-Albright syndrome.
5. Gigantism.
6. Pseudohypoparathyroidism.
7. Intracranial masses (hypothalamic region).

GENERALIZED INCREASED BONE DENSITY IN CHILDREN

1. Osteopetrosis.
2. Pyknodysostosis.
3. Renal osteodystrophy.
4. Lead poisoning.
5. Fluorosis.
6. Hypervitaminosis D.
7. Chronic hypervitaminosis A.
8. Caffey's disease.
9. Idiopathic hypercalcaemia of infancy.

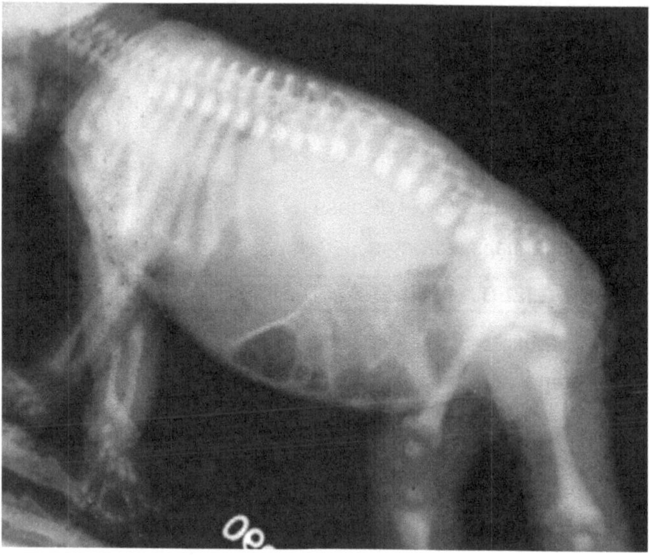

Figure 8.3: Radiograph showing generalized increased bone density in a case of hypervitaminosis D

PEDIATRIC TUMORS METASTASIZING TO BONE

1. Neuroblastoma.
2. Leukaemia.
3. Lymphoma.
4. Rhabdomyosarcoma.
5. Retinoblastoma.
6. Ewing's sarcoma.
7. Osteosarcoma.
8. Wilm's tumor.

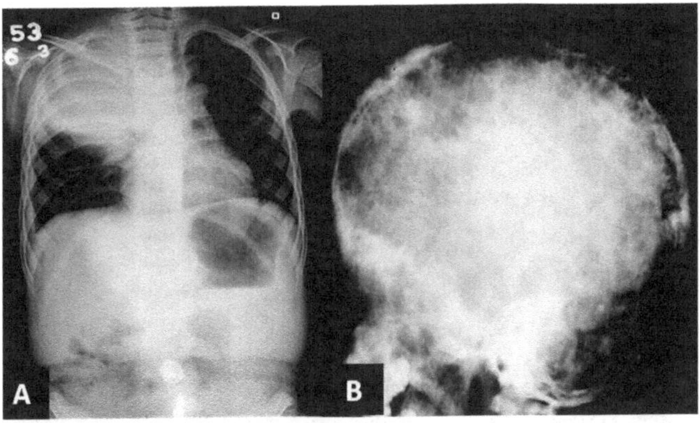

Figure 8.4: Radiograph showing (A) neuroblastoma metastases to the paraspinal region and vertebra (B) neuroblastoma metastases in the skull

GENERALISED OSTEOPENIA

1. Malnutrition.
2. Osteoporosis.
3. Hyperparathyroidism.
4. Leukaemia.
5. Rickets.

ERLENMEYER FLASK DEFORMITY

1. Pyle's disease (metaphyseal dysplasia).
2. Craniometaphyseal dysplasia.
3. Osteopetrosis.
4. Thalassaemia.
5. Gaucher's disease.
6. Niemann-Pick disease.
7. Lead poisoning.

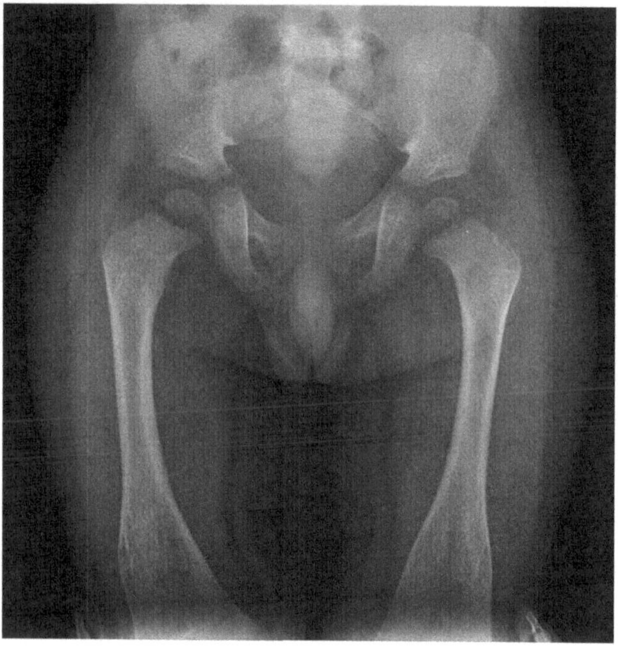

Figure 8.5: X-ray of pelvis including both femora showing widening of ischiopubic rami and Erlenmayer flask deformity of both femora in a case of Pyle's metaphyseal dysplasia

SOLITARY COLLAPSED VERTEBRA

1. Eosinophilic granuloma.
2. Infection.
3. Trauma.
4. Metastasis.

5. Lymphoma.
6. Benign tumors–Hemangioma, giant cell tumor, aneurysmal bone cyst.

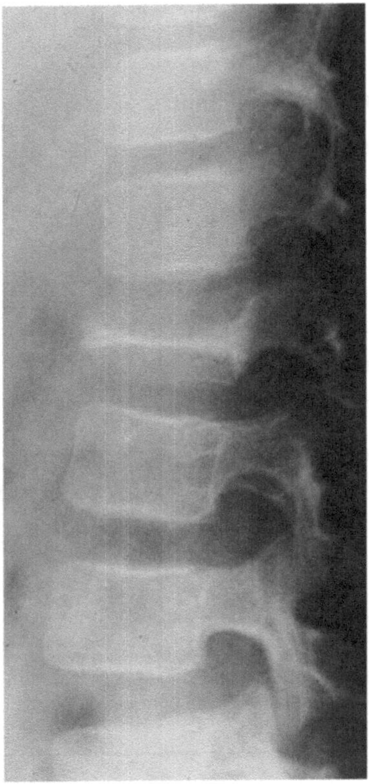

Figure 8.6: X-ray spine showing solitary collapsed vertebra in a case of eosinophilic granuloma

INCREASED DENSITY OF A HEMITHORAX

With Central Mediastinum

1. Consolidation.
2. Pleural effusion in a supine radiograph.
3. Mesothelioma.

Contralateral Mediastinal Shift

1. Pleural effusion.
2. Diaphragmatic hernia.

Ipsilateral Mediastinal Shift

1. Collapse.
2. Post-pneumonectomy.
3. Pulmonary agenesis.
4. Pulmonary hypoplasia.

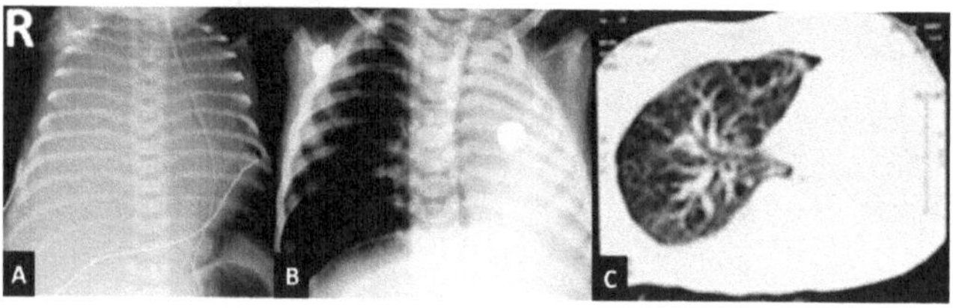

Figure 8.7: Chest radiograph showing (A) opaque right hemithorax with contralateral mediastinal shift (B,C) opaque left hemithorax in a case of left lung agenesis

PNEUMATOCELES

1. Infections – Staph. aureus, Streptococcus pneumoniae, E. coli, Klebsiella pneumoniae, Haemophilus influenzae, Pneumocystis carinii, Legionella pneumophilia.
2. Traumatic.
3. Following treatment for lung metastasis.

SOLITARY PULMONARY NODULE

1. Infective - Granulomas – tuberculoma, histoplasmoma.
   - Pneumococcal pneumonia.
   - Hydatid cyst.
2. Congenital – Sequestration, bronchogenic cyst.
3. Benign neoplasms – Adenoma, hamartoma.
4. Malignant neoplasms – Metastasis, lung malignancy (less common in children).
5. Vascular – Pulmonary infarction, haematoma, arteriovenous malformation.

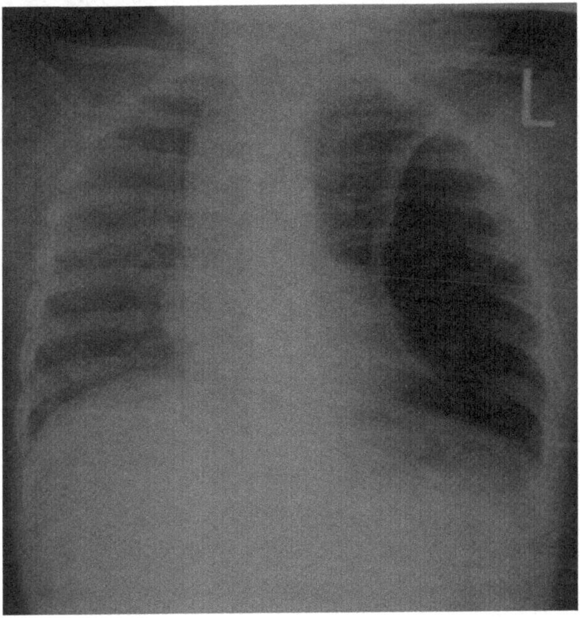

Figure 8.8: Chest radiograph showing large pneumatoceles in left lung field in a case of staphylococcal pneumonia

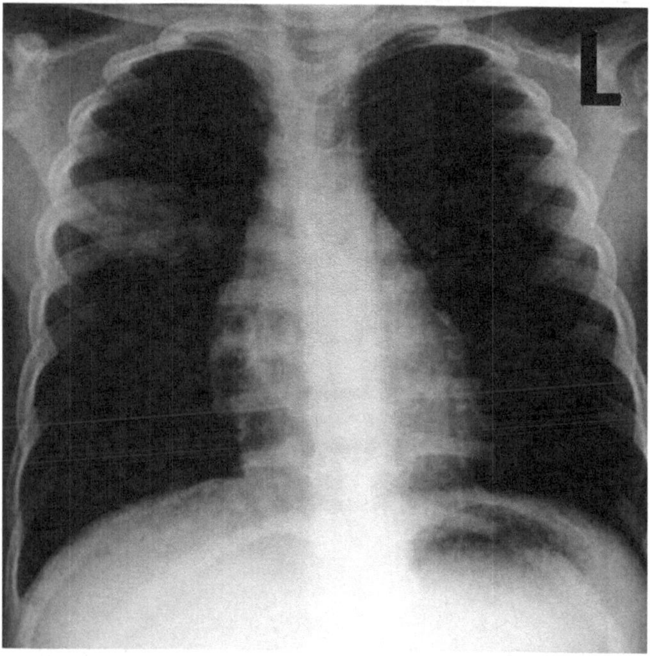

Figure 8.9: Chest radiograph showing consolidation with air-bronchogram in right upper and mid-zones

OPACITY WITH AIR-BRONCHOGRAM

1. Infective – pneumonia.
2. Inflammatory.
3. Malignancy – lymphoma, lymphosarcoma, alveolar cell carcinoma.

UNILATERAL ELEVATED HEMIDIAPHRAGM

Causes Above the Diaphragm

1. Phrenic nerve palsy.
2. Collapse.
3. Pulmonary infarction.
4. Hemiplegia.
5. Pleural pathologies.

Diaphragmatic Causes

1. Eventration.

Causes Below the Diaphragm

1. Gaseous distension of stomach.
2. Subphrenic abscess.
3. Pancreatitis.

SCOLIOSIS

Decubitus Film on Dependent Side

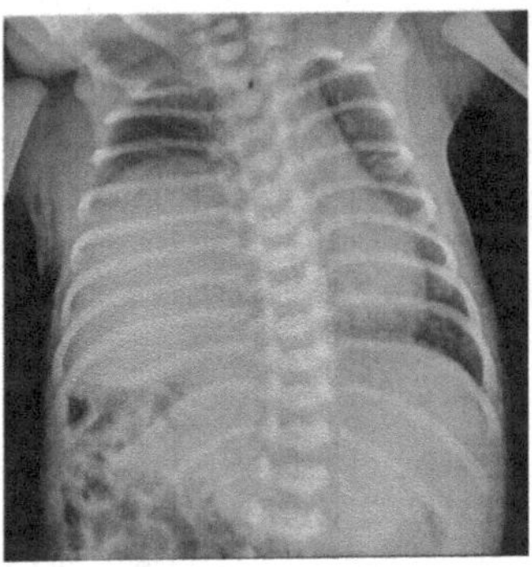

Figure 8.10: Chest radiograph showing elevated right hemidiaphragm in case of eventration

INTRA-ABDOMINAL CALCIFICATIONS IN NEWBORN

1. Meconium peritonitis.
2. Meconium ileus.
3. Bowel atresia.
4. Intestinal obstruction–imperforate anus, Hirschsprung's disease.

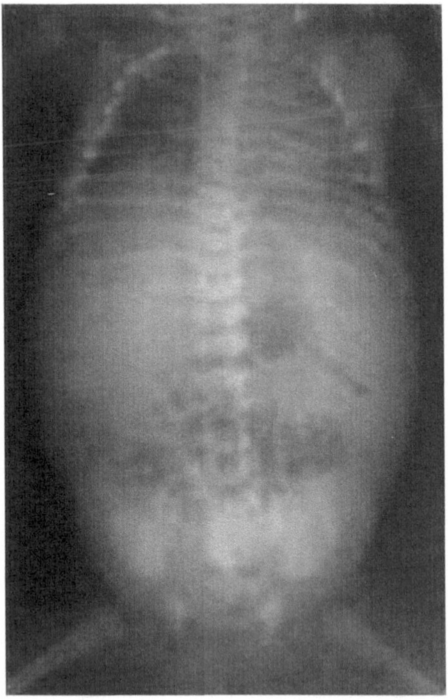

Figure 8.11: Radiograph of abdomen of a classical case of meconium peritonitis

GAS IN THE PORTAL VEINS

1. Necrotizing enterocolitis.
2. Umbilical vein catheterization.
3. Erythroblastosis fetalis.
4. Mesenteric ischemia.
5. Air embolism post double contrast barium enema study.

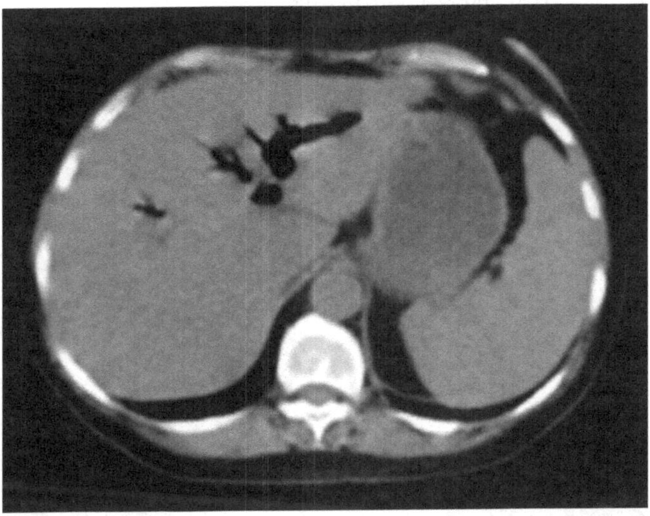

Figure 8.12: Axial non-contrast CT abdomen showing gas in the portal veins in a case of mesenteric ischemia

ADRENAL CALCIFICATION

1. Neuroblastoma.
2. Adrenal haemorrhage.
3. Wolman's disease.
4. Ganglioneuroma.
5. Addison's disease.
6. Post-infective–tuberculosis, histoplasmosis.
7. Rarely in phaeochromocytoma.

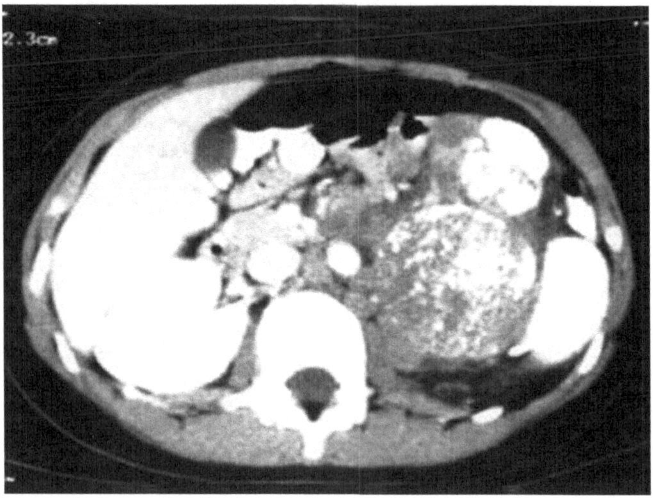

Figure 8.13: Axial contrast CT abdomen showing calcification in left adrenal gland in a case of neuroblastoma

MACROCEPHALY IN INFANCY

1. Hydrocephalus.
2. Neurofibromatosis.
3. Mucopolysaccharidosis.
4. Alexander's disease.
5. Canavan's disease.
6. Hydranencephaly.
7. Subdural hematoma.
8. Progeria.

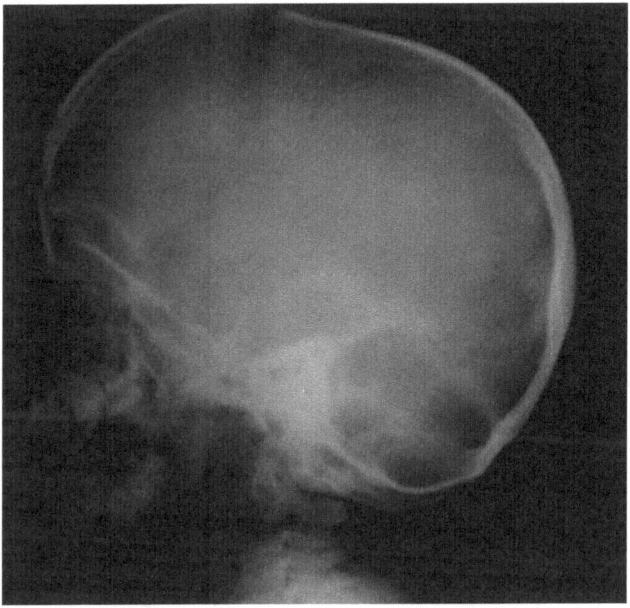

Figure 8.14: X-ray skull showing macrocephaly in a case of mucopolysaccharidosis

WIDENED CRANIAL SUTURES

Sutures are said to be widened if they are >10 mm at birth; >3 mm at 2 years of age; and > 2 mm at 3 years of age.

Causes of Widening of Sutures:

1. Hydrocephalus.
2. Intracranial tumor.
3. Neuroblastoma.
4. Leukaemia.
5. Lymphoma.
6. Rickets.
7. Prematurity.
8. Hypothyroidism.
9. Bony dysplasias.

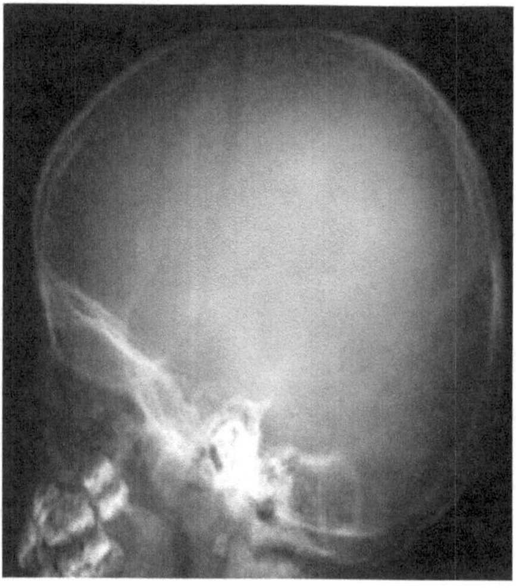

Figure 8.15: X-ray skull showing widened sutures in a case of premature neonate

SYNDROMES ASSOCIATED WITH HYDROCEPHALUS

1. Achondroplasia.
2. Crouzon's syndrome.
3. Osteopetrosis.
4. Soto's syndrome.
5. Lissencephaly.
6. Mucopolysaccharidosis.
7. Thanatophoric dysplasia.
8. Metachromatic leukodystrophy.

NORMAL INTRACRANIAL CALCIFICATION

1. Pineal gland.
2. Choroid plexus.
3. Dura.
4. Basal ganglia.
5. Habenular commissure.
6. Dentate nuclei.
7. Parasellar ligaments.
8. Arachnoid granulations.

BASAL GANGLIA CALCIFICATION

1. Normal.
2. Metabolic–Mitochondrial disorders, Fahr's disease, Cockayne's syndrome.
3. Endocrine–Hypoparathyroidism, pseudohypoparathyroidism, hypothyroidism.
4. Infections.
5. Hypoxia.
6. Carbon monoxide poisoning.

7. Lead intoxication.
8. Post-chemo/radiotherapy.

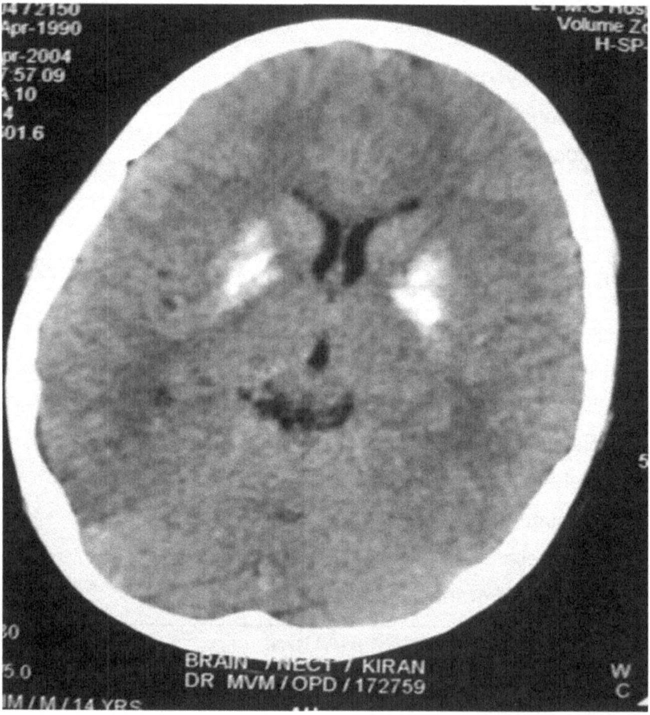

Figure 8.16: Axial NCCT head showing bilateral basal ganglia calcification

ENHANCEMENT OF MENINGES

1. Infection.
2. Tumor – Metastases, leukaemia, lymphoma, germinoma, medulloblastoma, LCH.
3. Sarcoidosis.
4. Subacute stage of subarachnoid haemorrhage.
5. Subacute infarct.
5. Sturge-Weber syndrome.
6. Venous thrombosis.
7. Extramedullary haematopoiesis.

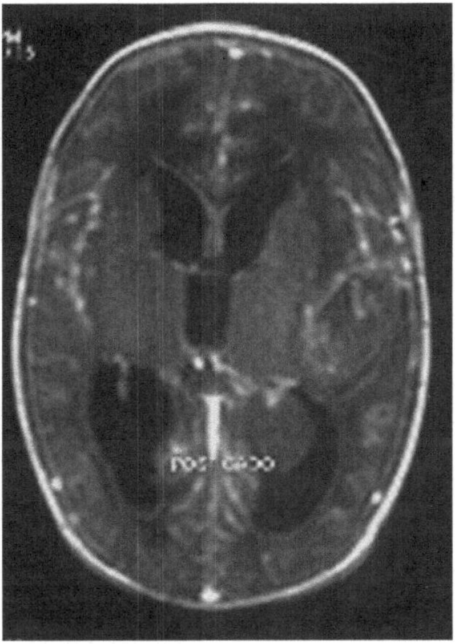

Figure 8.17: Contrast MRI image showing enhancement of meninges in a case of pyogenic meningitis

RING ENHANCING LESIONS IN BRAIN

1. Neurocysticercosis.
2. Tuberculoma.
3. Metastases.
4. Abscesses.
5. Lymphoma.
6. Demyelination.
7. Glioma.
8. Subacute infarct.
9. Subacute hematoma.
10. Demyelination.

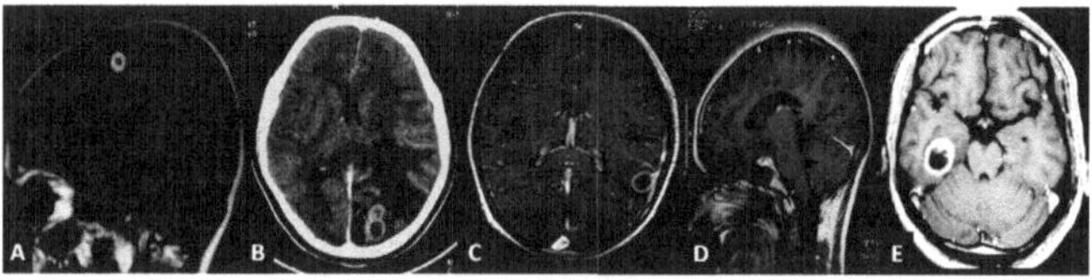

Figure 8.18: Ring enhancing lesions (A) neurocysticercosis (B) tuberculoma (C) abscess (D) demyelination and (E) DNET

MR BRAIN T1 HYPERINTENSE BASAL GANGLIA

1. Intracranial haemorrhage.
2. Wilson's disease.
3. Japanese encephalitis.
4. Long-term total parenteral nutrition due to manganese deposition.
5. Haemorrhagic infarction.
6. Calcification.
7. Neurofibromatosis Type I.
8. Profound hypoxia.
9. Chronic liver disease.

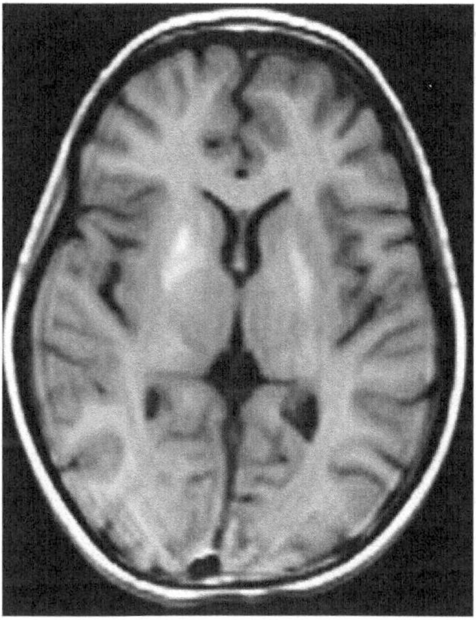

Figure 8.19: Axial T1-weighted MR image showing hyperintensity in bilateral basal ganglia in case of hyperalimentation

MR BRAIN T2 HYPERINTENSE BASAL GANGLIA

1. Hypoxia.
2. Venous infarction.
3. Wilson's disease.
4. Huntington disease.
5. Mitochondrial diseases.
6. Extrapontine myelinolysis.
7. Carbon monoxide poisoning.
8. Hypoglycemia.
9. Cyanide poisoning.
10. Methanol poisoning.
11. Kernicterus.

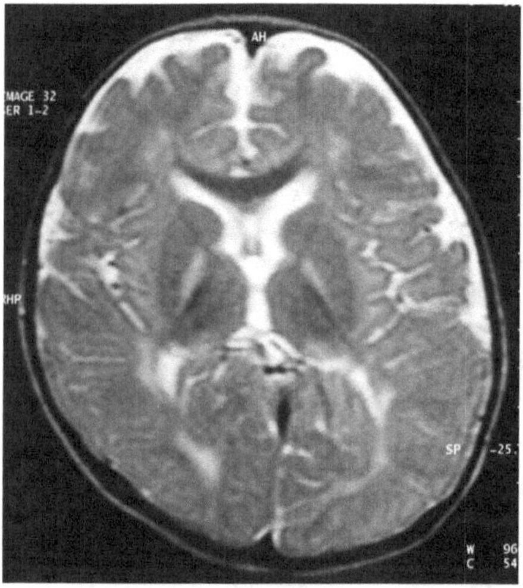

Figure 8.20: Axial T2-weighted MR image showing hyperintensity in bilateral globus pallidi in a case of Kernicterus

MR BRAIN T2 HYPERINTENSITY IN BILATERAL THALAMI

1. Lacunar infarcts.
2. Venous infarct.
3. Artery of percheron infarct.
4. Severe anoxia.
5. Japanese encephalitis.
6. Carbon monoxide poisoning.
7. Wernicke's encephalopathy.
8. Mitochondria cytopathies.
9. ADEM.

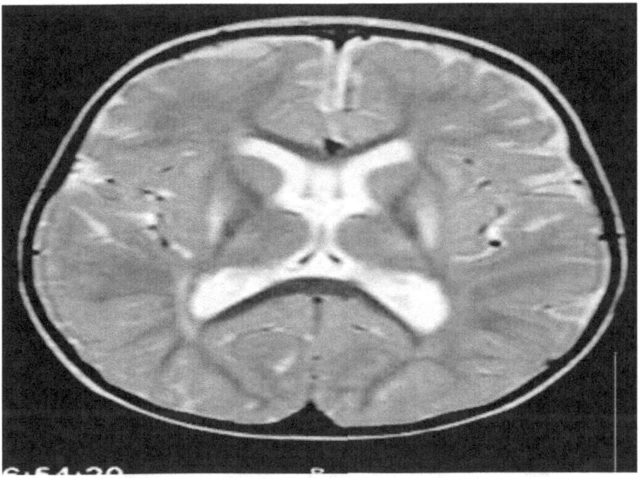

Figure 8.21: Axial T2-weighted MR image showing hyperintensity in bilateral basal ganglia and thalami in case of anoxic insult in a term neonate

MULTIPLE WORMIAN BONES

Definition: Intrasutural bones considered abnormal if large (greater than 6 mm) and multiple (more than 10).

Causes

1. Pyknodysostosis.
2. Osteogenesis imperfecta.
3. Rickets.
4. Kinky-Hair syndrome.
5. Cleido-cranial dysostosis.
6. Hypophophatasia.
7. Hypothyroidism.
8. Down's syndrome.
9. Otopalatodigital syndrome.
10. Progeria.
11. Pachydermoperiostosis.
12. Idiopathic.

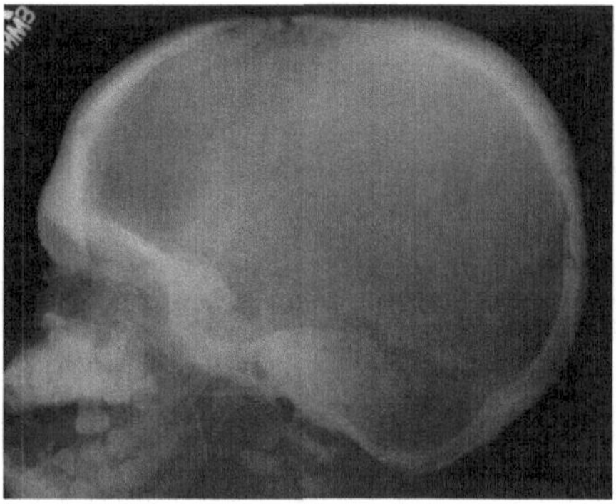

Figure 8.22: Skull X-ray showing widened sutures and wormian bones in a case of hypothyroidism

HAIR-ON-END SKULL VAULT

1. Hemolytic anaemias.
2. Neoplastic – hemangioma, meningioma, metastasis.
3. Cyanotic heart disease.
4. Iron deficiency anaemia.

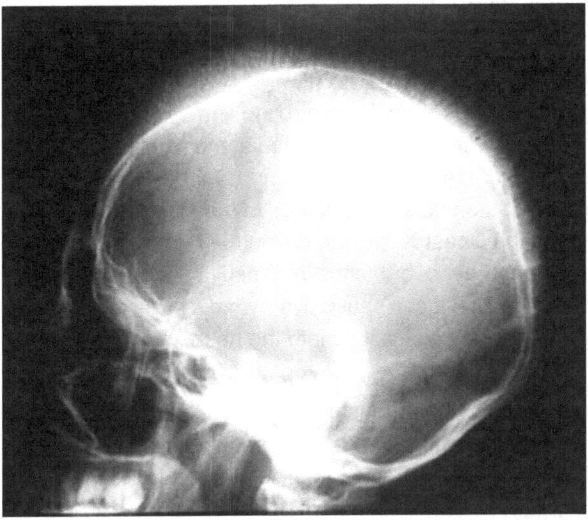

Figure 8.23: Skull X-ray showing hair-on-end appearance in a case of thalassemia

TUBES AND LINES

Nasogastric tube: The tip of the NG tube should be positioned at least 10 cm caudal to location of the gastroesophageal junction. The tip of a nasoduodenal feeding tube should be inserted at least 10-12 cm into the small bowel.

Endotracheal tube: The tip of an ET tube in the neutral position of the neck should be 5-7 cm above the carina. The location can vary approximately 2 cm in the caudal or cephalad directions with neck flexion and extension, respectively. When the carina is not visible, the tip of the ET tube should be approximately at the level of the medial ends of the clavicle.

Tracheostomy: The tip of the tracheostomy tube should be half way between the stoma and the carina, at the level of the D3 vertebra.

Central venous line: The tip of the line should be distal to the last venous valve, which is located at the junction of the internal jugular and the subclavian veins. On the Chest X-ray, the position of the valve corresponds to the inner aspect of the first rib. On the Chest X-ray, the cavoatrial junction corresponds to the lower border of bronchus intermedius. If the line tip reaches the right atrium, it can cause dysrhythmia or result in injection of undiluted toxic medications into the heart.

Pulmonary artery (Swan-Ganz) catheter: The tip of the Swan-Ganz catheter must not be more than 1 cm lateral to the mediastinal margin. The catheter should not extend beyond the pulmonary hilum on the CXR; else, it should be retracted.

Pacemaker: The single-lead pacemaker is the most basic type and is positioned with its tip in the right ventricular apex. An atrioventricular two-lead sequential pacemaker has one electrode in the right atrium and the other at the right ventricular apex. Sometimes a third lead is placed in the coronary sinus to pace the left ventricle. Twiddler's syndrome is a rare disorder in which twisting of the lead occurs either due to the patient's manipulation or spontaneously.

Umbilical venous catheter: Tip should be approximately at the level of D8-D9 vertebrae in the IVC at the level of diaphragm. It lies on the right side on the anteroposterior radiograph. On the lateral CXR, it lies anteriorly. There should be no coiling, bend, or kink in the catheter.

Umbilical artery catheter: The umbilical artery catheter should be at the level of the D6-D10 vertebrae (high position) or at the level of the L3-4 vertebrae (low position) to ensure that its tip is away from the origins of vessels supplying vital organs (the carotids in the high position and the renal vessels in the low position). In contrast to the umbilical venous catheter, the umbilical artery catheter dips initially before it takes a path parallel to the spine on the left side. On a lateral X-ray, it lies posteriorly.

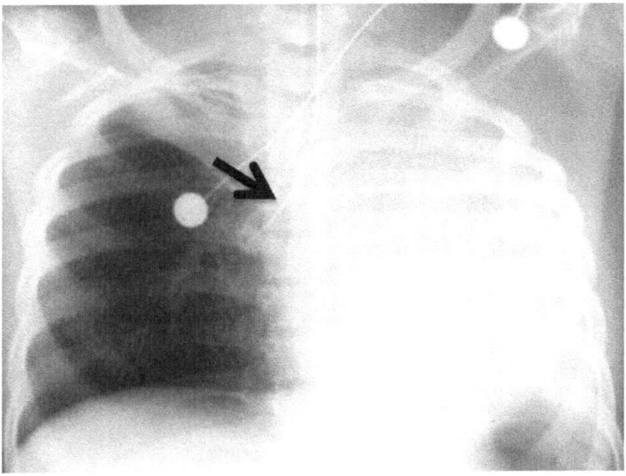

Figure 8.24: Chest radiograph showing malpositioned endotracheal tube (arrow) placed in right bronchus resulting in collapse of left lung

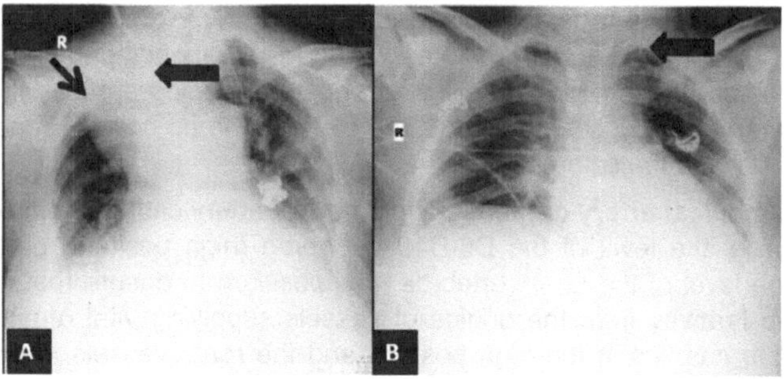

Figure 8.25: Chest radiographs showing malpositioned central line (arrowhead) (A) leading to mediastinal hematoma (arrow) and (B) tip misplaced in left jugular vein

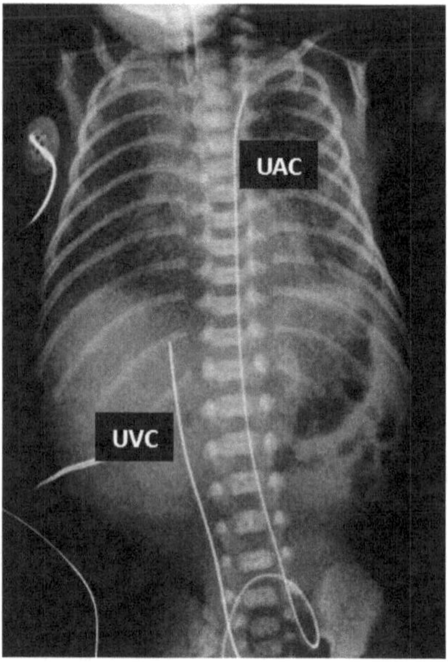

Figure 8.26: Neonatal radiograph showing malpositioned umbilical venous catheter (UVC) lying below the level of diaphragm and malpositioned umbilical artery catheter (UAC) tip placed in subclavian artery

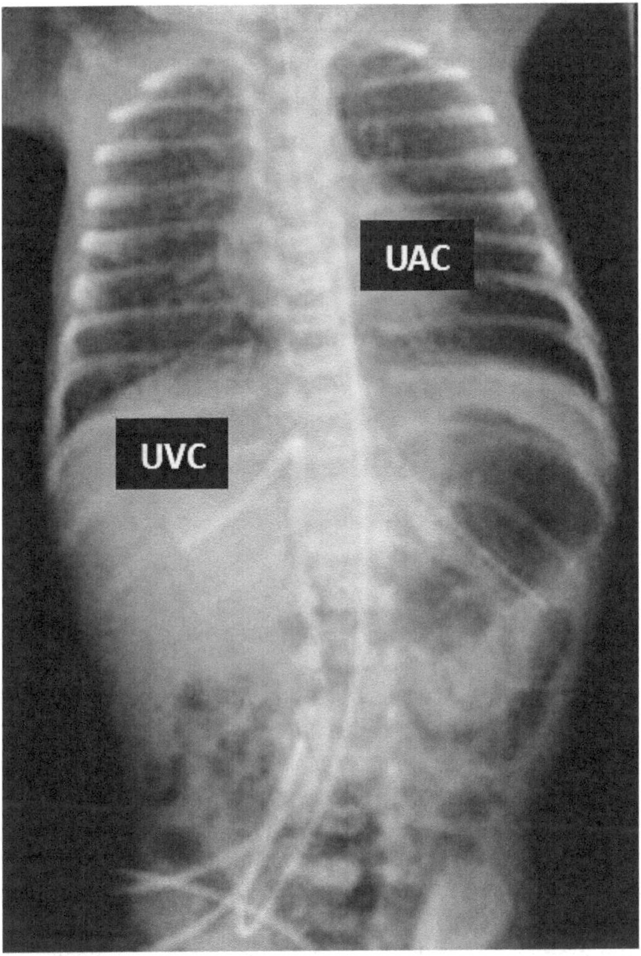

Figure 8.27: Neonatal radiograph showing malpositioned umbilical venous catheter (UVC) lying in right portal vein and normal position of umbilical artery catheter (UAC)

FOREIGN BODY IN AIRWAY AND ESOPHAGUS

Coins in the esophagus are round in appearance on the frontal view whereas coins in the trachea are usually seen on end and are linear in shape.

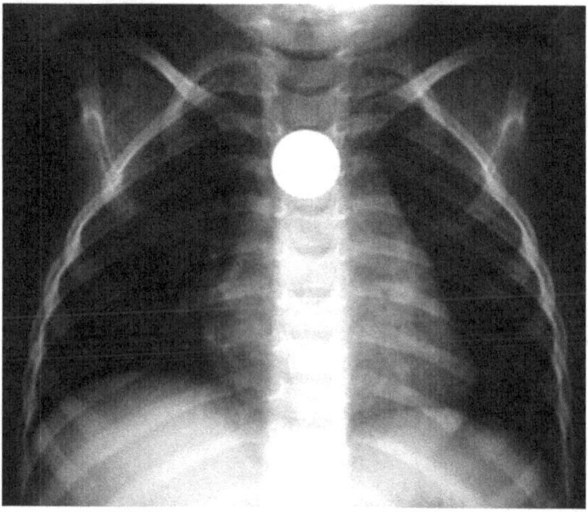

Figure 8.28: Chest radiograph showing foreign body (coin) in esophagus

- Chest X-ray will be normal in ~35% (range 30-40%) of patients.
- Unilateral emphysema or atelectasis is the most common findings.

Opaque foreign bodies on X-ray: Glass of all types; most metallic objects (except aluminum); most animal bones and some fish bones; some foods; some soil fragments, sand, gravel, and mineral fragments; some medications and poisons.

Nonopaque materials on X-ray: Most foods and medicines; most fish bones; most wood, splinters, thorns of all types; most plastics; most aluminum objects.

NEPHROCALCINOSIS

Medullary Nephrocalcinosis

1. Hyperparathyroidism.
2. Renal tubular acidosis.
3. Medullary sponge kidney.
4. Preterm infants.
5. Primary hyperoxaluria.
6. Sarcoidosis.
7. Milk-Alkali syndrome.
8. Idiopathic hypercalciuria.

Cortical Nephrocalcinosis

1. Acute cortical necrosis.
2. Chronic glomerulonephritis.
3. Chronic transplant rejection.

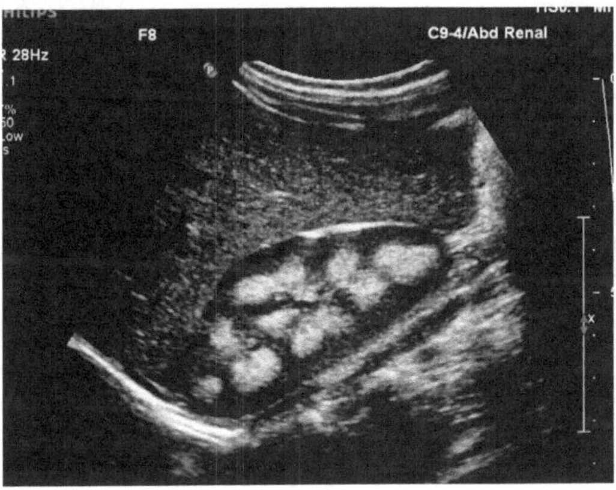

Figure 8.29: Ultrasound image showing hyperechoic shadows with acoustic shadowing in a case of medullary nephrocalcinosis

LARYNGOTRACHEOBRONCHITIS

X-Ray Findings:

Steeple sign – Seen on AP radiographs of the neck or chest and neck demonstrates uniform narrowing of the subglottic airway; also referred to as a wine bottle sign.

Distension of the hypopharynx is also seen due to the patient's attempt at decreasing airway resistance.

Lateral radiograph of the upper airway will show a normal epiglottis and narrowing of the subglottic region.

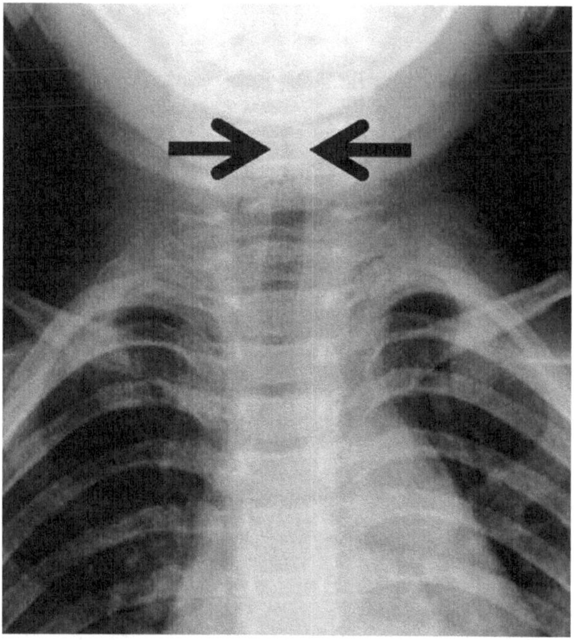

Figure 8.30: Chest radiograph showing narrowing in subglottic region suggestive of steeple sign in a case of layngotracheobronchitis

EPIGLOTTITIS

X-Ray Findings:

Lateral radiograph demonstrates thickening of epiglottis and aryepiglottic folds which is called thumb sign. Hypopharynx may be over-distended.

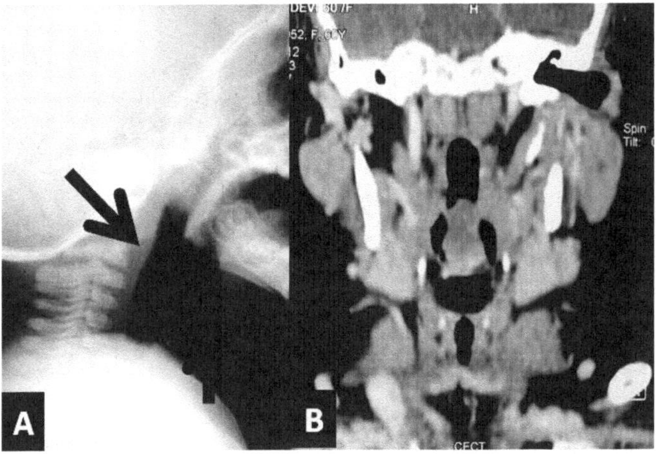

Figure 8.31: (A) X-ray soft tissue neck showing thickening of epiglottis and dilated hypopharynx (B) Coronal CT image showing epiglottis thickening in a case of epiglottitis

BATTERED BABY SYNDROME

Fractures:

Bucket handle or Corner fractures.

Posterior rib fractures.

Fractures of acromion, sternum, spinous process.

Skull fractures – Occipital impression fractures, fractures crossing sutures.

Fracture in different stage of healing.

CNS Injuries

Subdural hemorrhage.

Subarachnoid hemorrhage.

Diffuse axonal injury.

Cerebral edema.

Visceral Injury

Perforation or hematoma.

Liver and pancreatic laceration.

Adrenal hemorrhage.

Retinal hemorrhage.

Spinal cord compression/injury.

Radiological Survey in Suspected Abuse

Chest AP and lateral.

Skull lateral.

Humerus.

Forearms.

Hands, Pelvis, Femurs, Lower legs, Ankle, Feet.

In children less than 12 months X-ray dorsolumbar spine lateral view and head CT.

In children less than 12 months and with neurological symptoms non-contrast head CT scan.

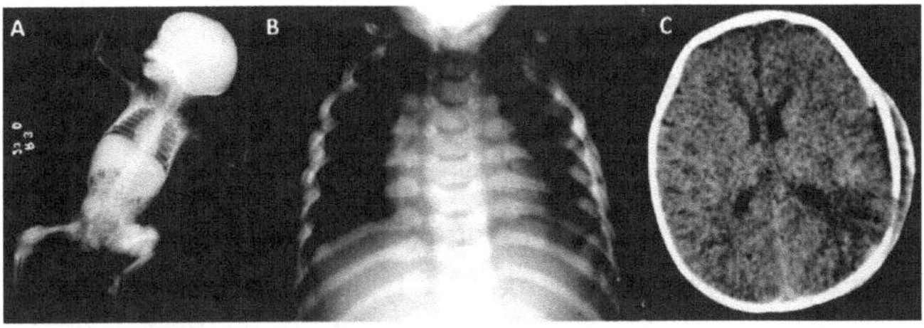

Figure 8.32: Three cases of child abuse (A) Trauma to right lower femur with calcified hematoma (B) Multiple rib fractures and fracture of left clavicle (C) NCCT head showing fracture skull with subdural and scalp hematoma

ADRENAL HEMORRHAGE

Extensive adrenal hemorrhage may occur at any age and under various circumstances such as severe stress as in surgery, sepsis, burns, hypotension, trauma, hemorrhagic diathesis and underlying conditions such as adenoma, cyst and tumour.

Ultrasound

Depending on the age of adrenal hematoma; it may show varied appearances on ultrasound. An early-stage hematoma appears solid with diffuse or inhomogeneous echogenicity. As liquefaction occurs, the mass demonstrates mixed echogenicity with a central hypoechoic region and eventually becomes completely anechoic and cyst-like.

Calcification may be seen in the later stages.

Colour Doppler shows absence of internal vascularity within the mass.

CT

Depending on the age of adrenal hematomas attenuation value in acute to subacute hematomas range from 50-90 HU. Over time, adrenal hematomas decrease in size and attenuation and most resolve completely. In later stages they may appear as adrenal cyst or may show calcification.

MRI

Depending on the age of adrenal hematomas; acute stage (less than 7 days): the hematoma typically appears isointense or slightly hypointense on T1 weighted images and markedly hypointense on T2 weighted images. In subacute stage (7 days to 7 weeks): the hematoma appears hyperintense on T1 and T2 weighted images and in chronic stage (after 7 weeks): a hypointense rim is present on T1 and T2 weighted images, which is attributed to hemosiderin deposition.

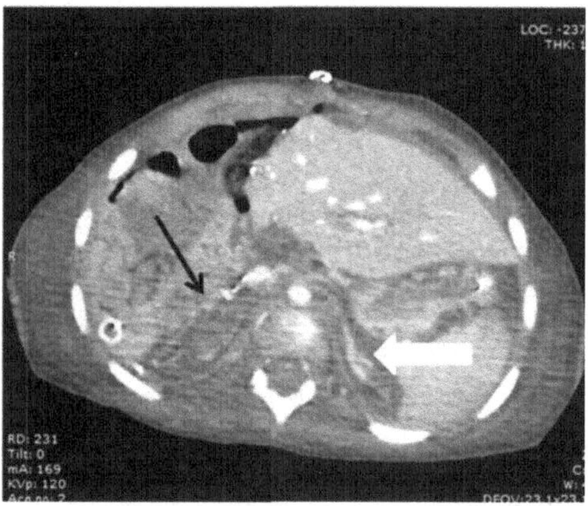

Figure 8.33: CECT abdomen showing right adrenal hemorrhage (arrow) and normal left adrenal gland (arrowhead)

Chapter 9

Brainstorming

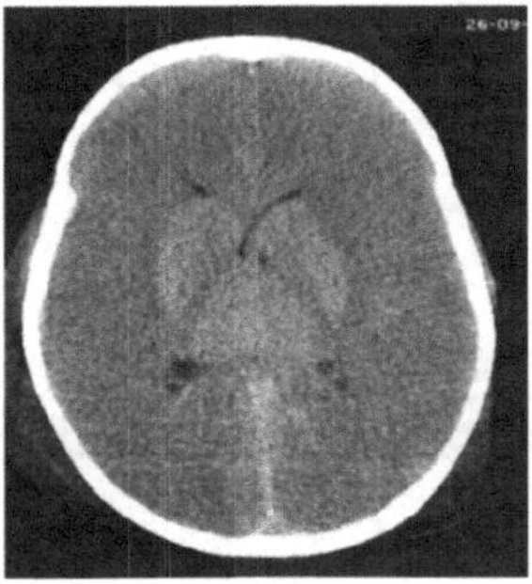

Figure 9.1

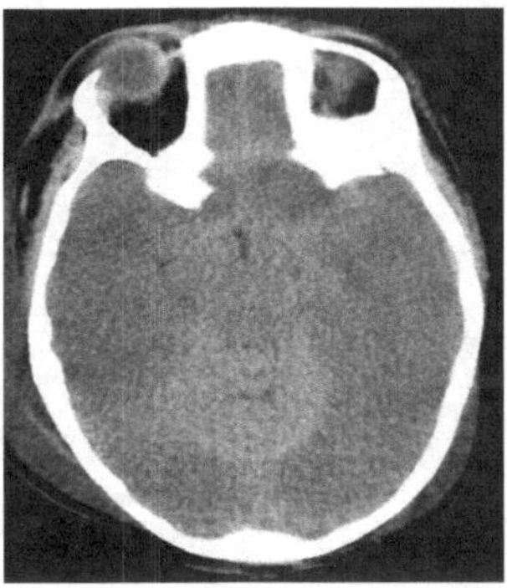

Figure 9.2

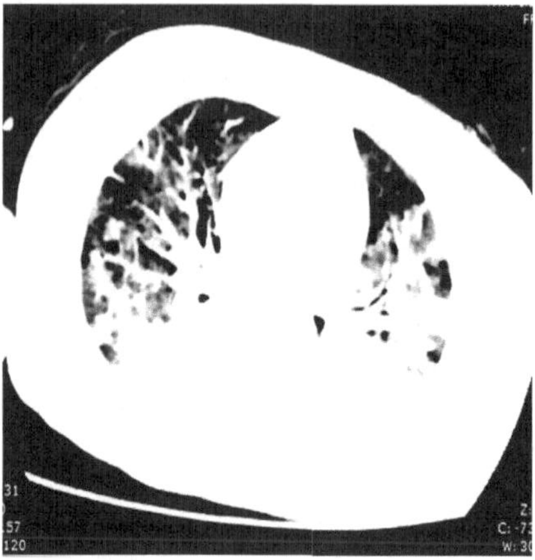

Figure 9.3

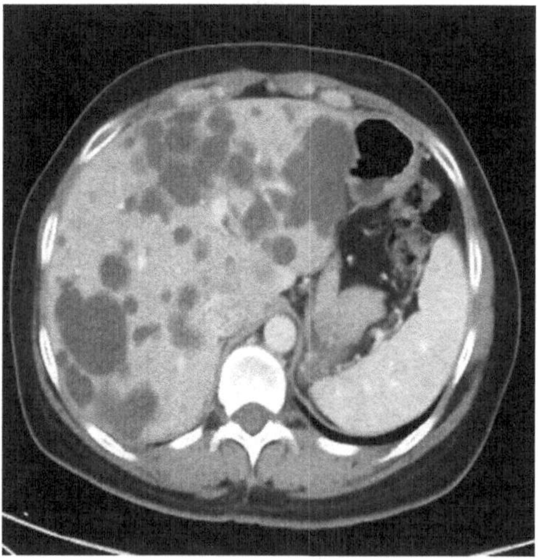

Figure 9.4

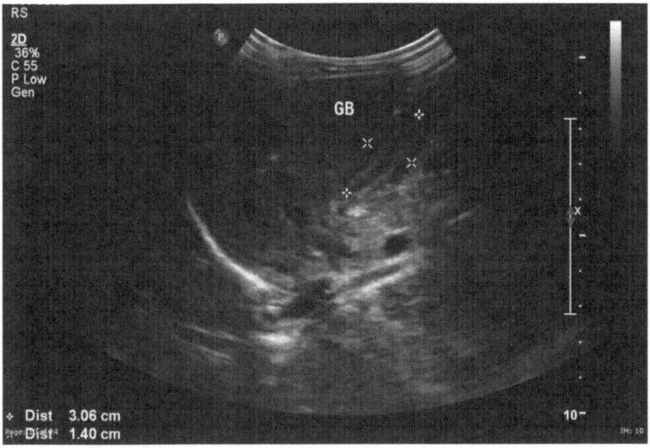

Figure 9.5

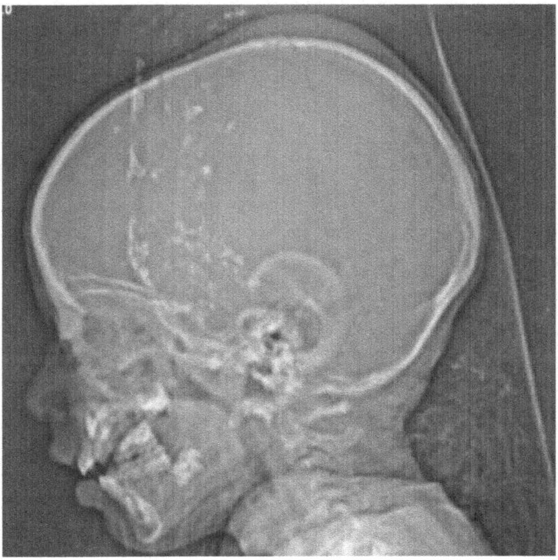

Figure 9.6

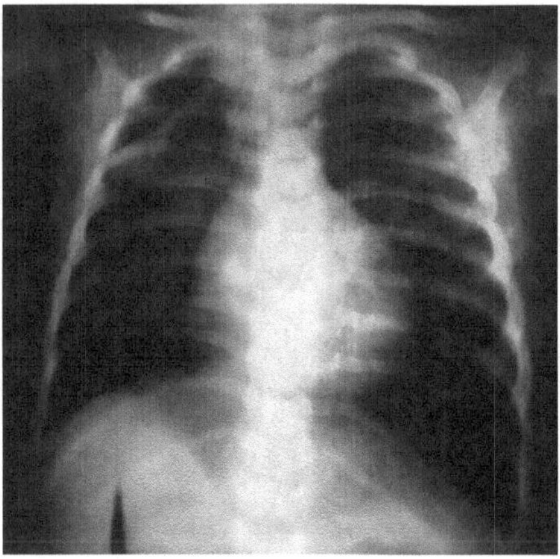

Figure 9.7

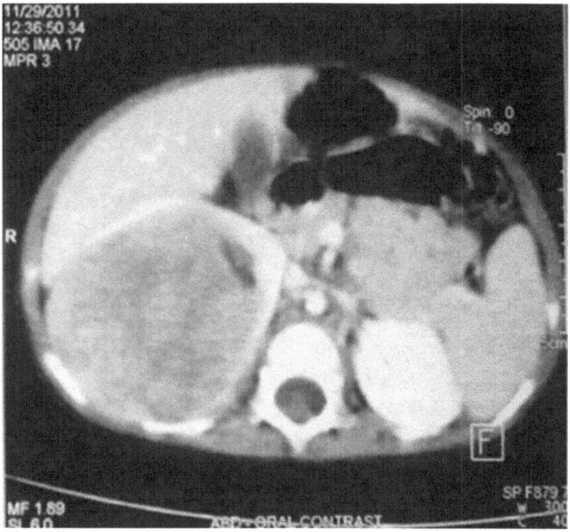

Figure 9.8

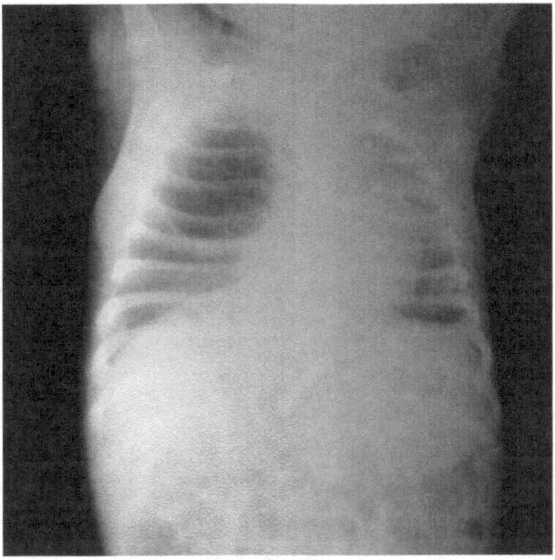

Figure 9.9

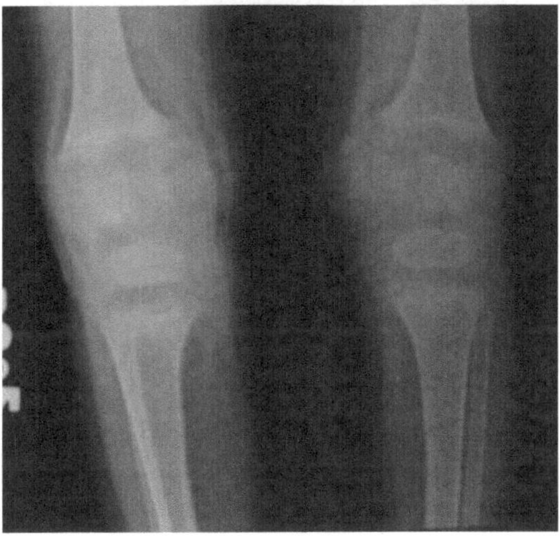

Figure 9.10

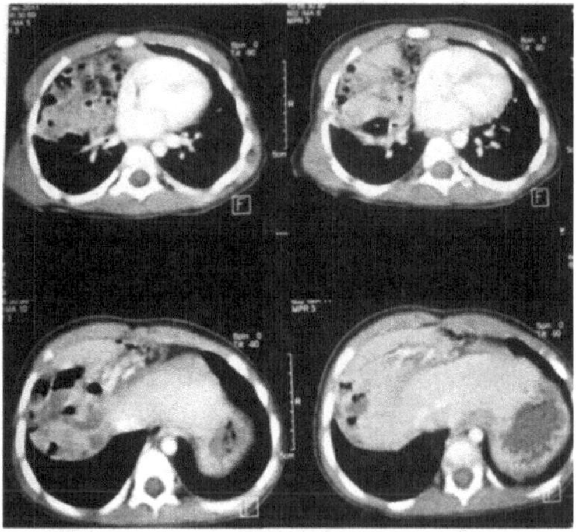

Figure 9.11

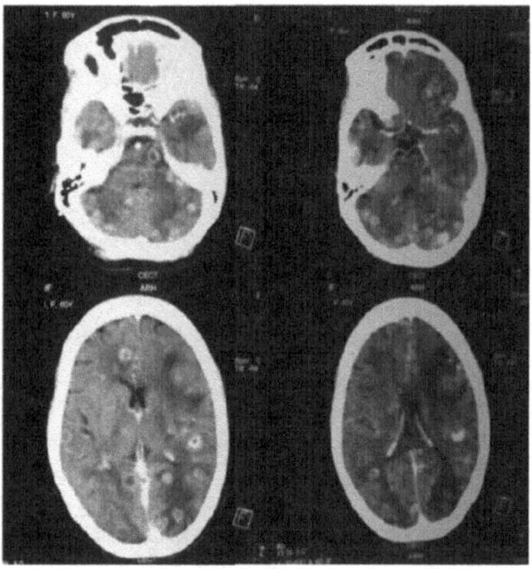

Figure 9.12

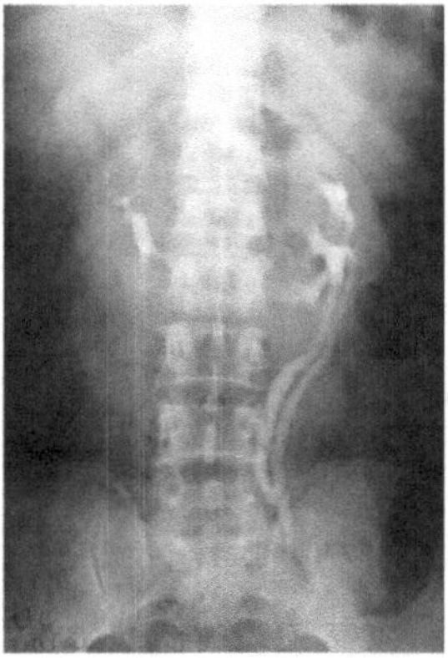

Figure 9.13

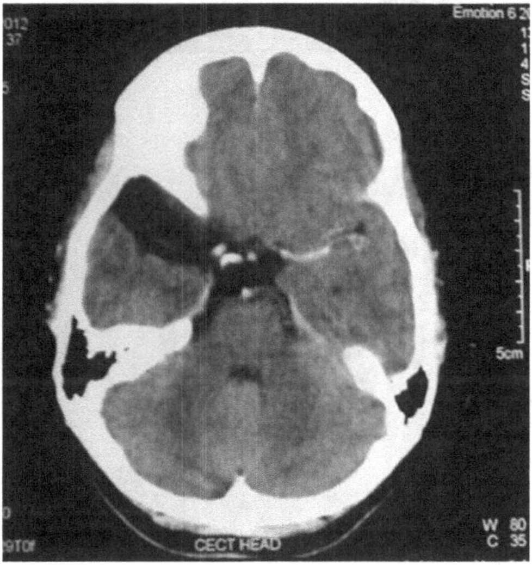

Figure 9.14

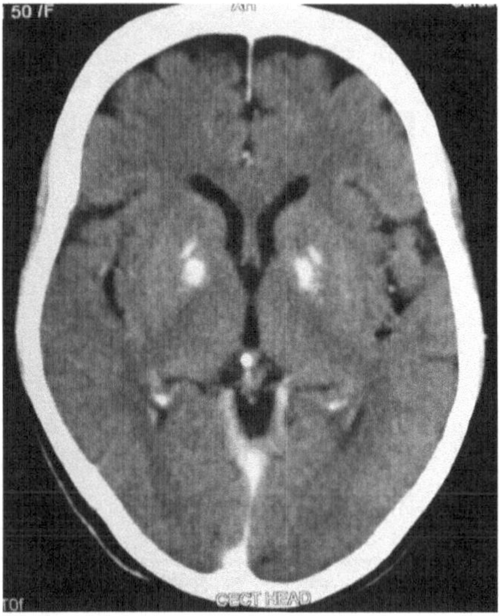

Figure 9.15

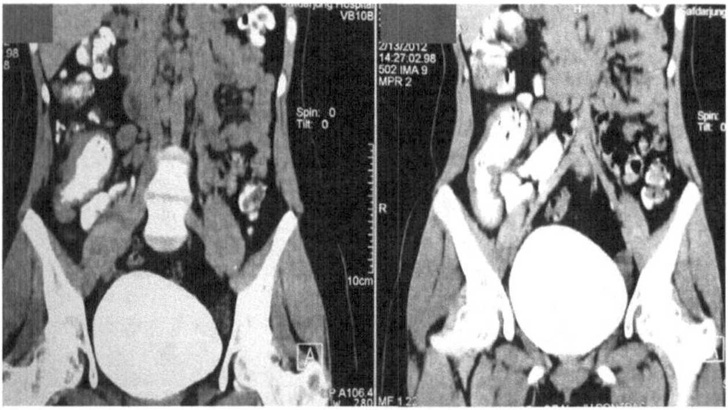

Figure 9.16

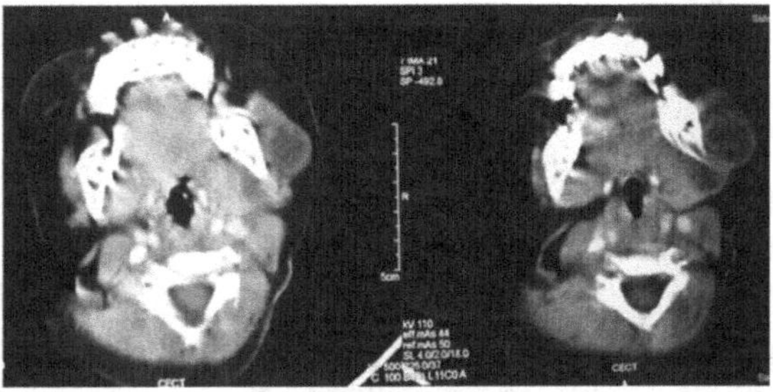

Figure 9.17

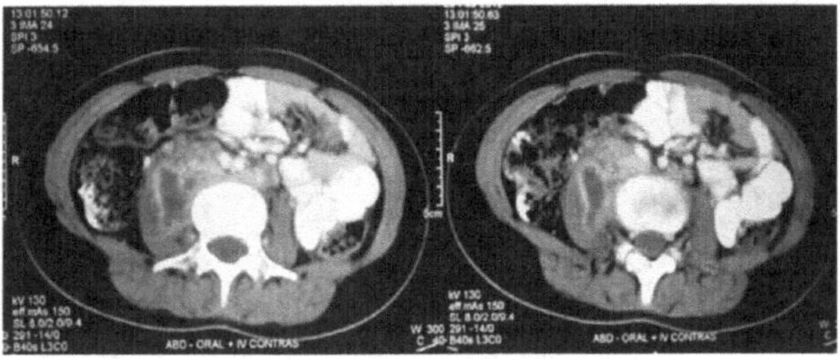

Figure 9.18

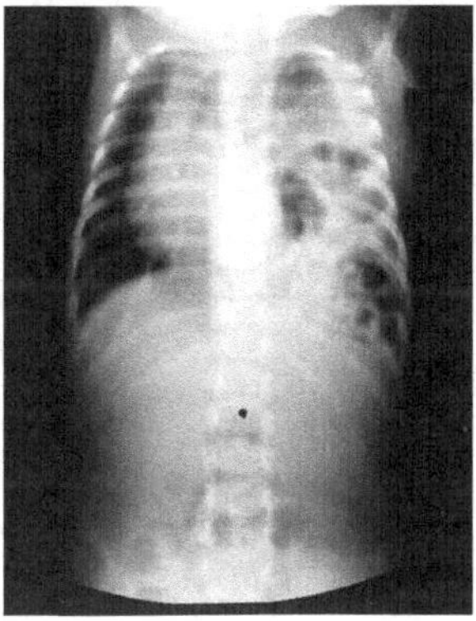

Figure 9.19

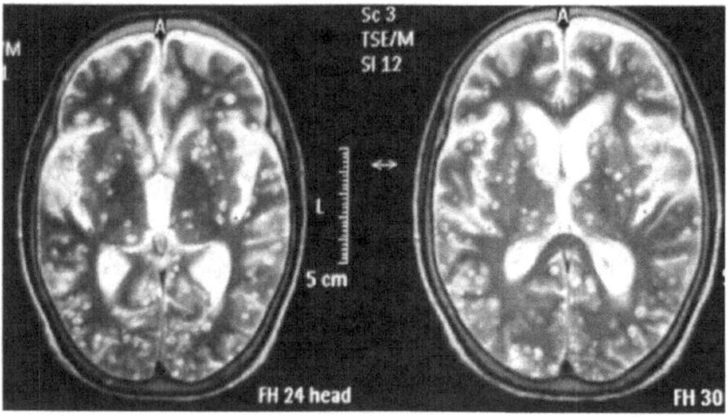

Figure 9.20

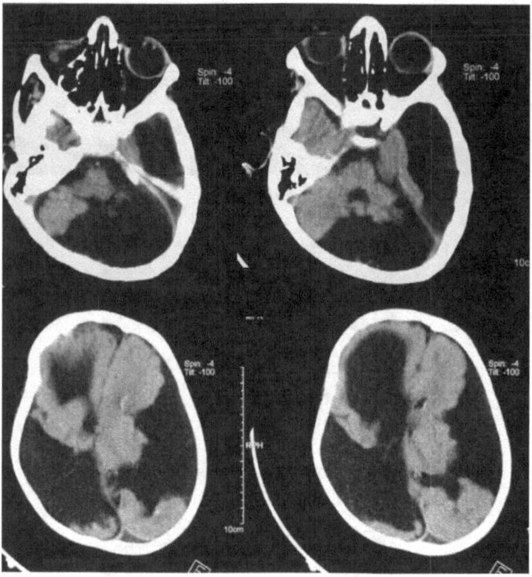

Figure 9.21

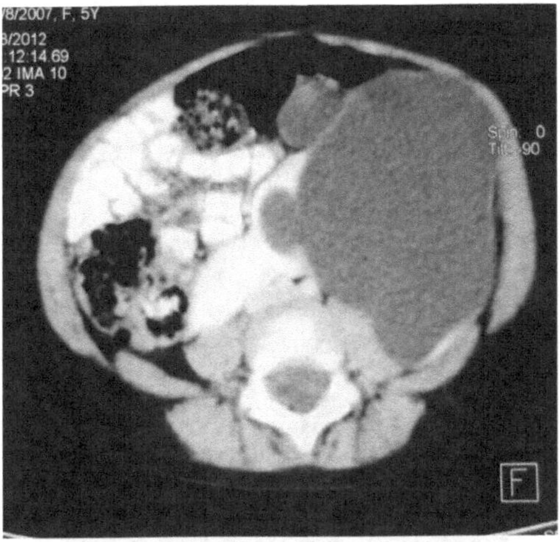

Figure 9.22

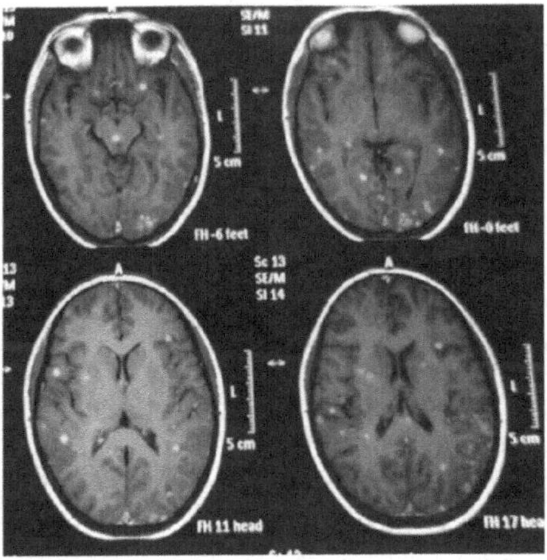

Figure 9.23

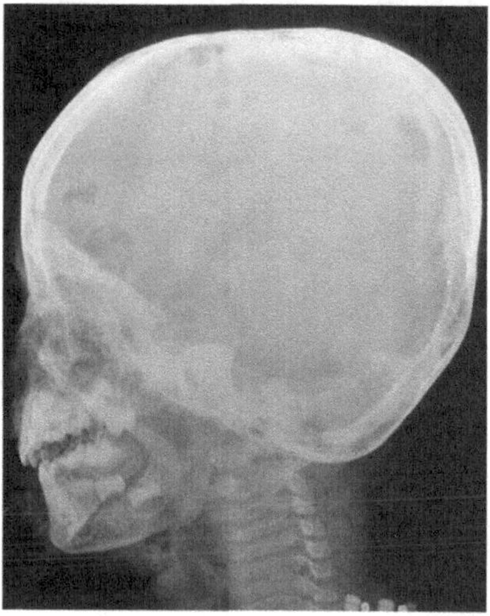

Figure 9.24

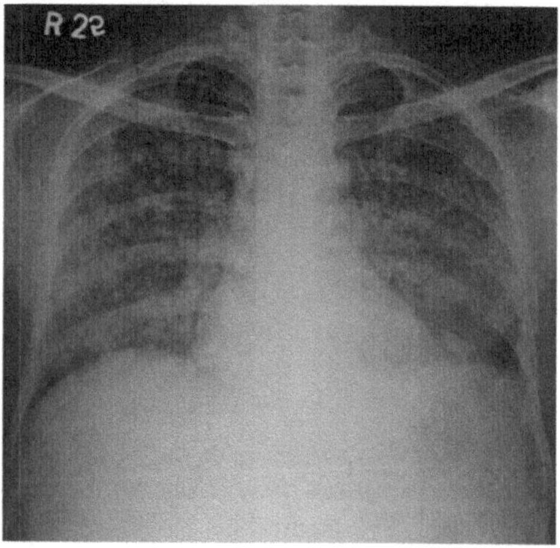

Figure 9.25

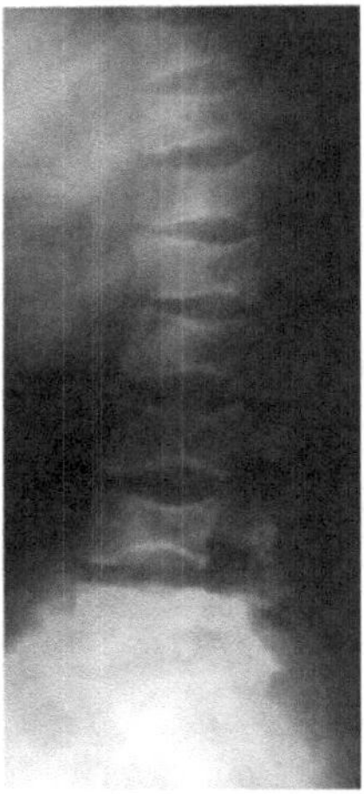

Figure 9.26

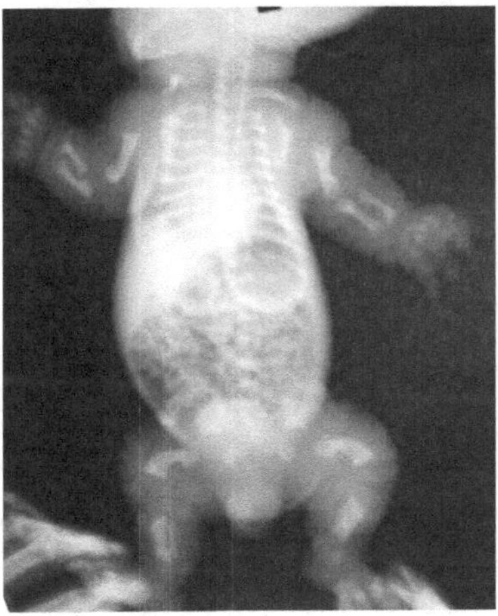

Figure 9.27

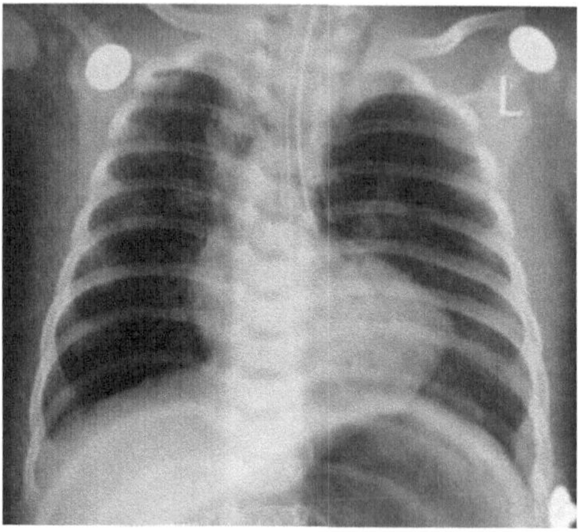

Figure 9.28

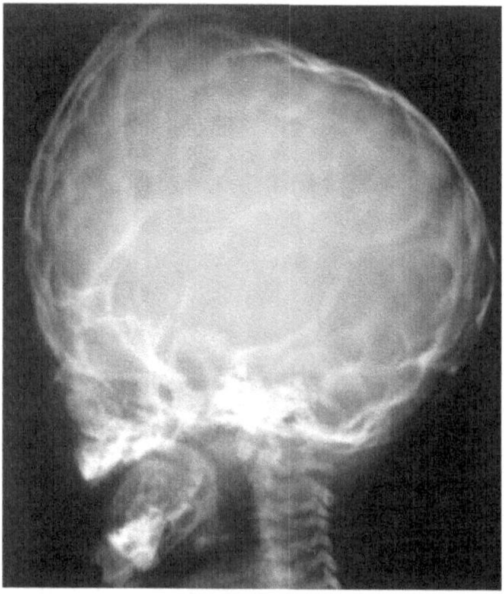

Figure 9.29

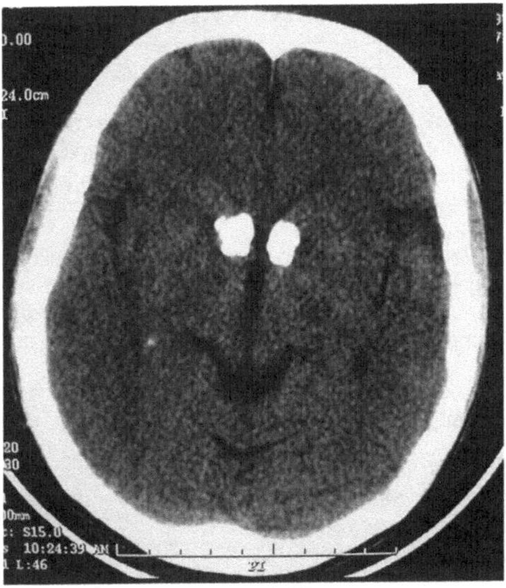

Figure 9.30

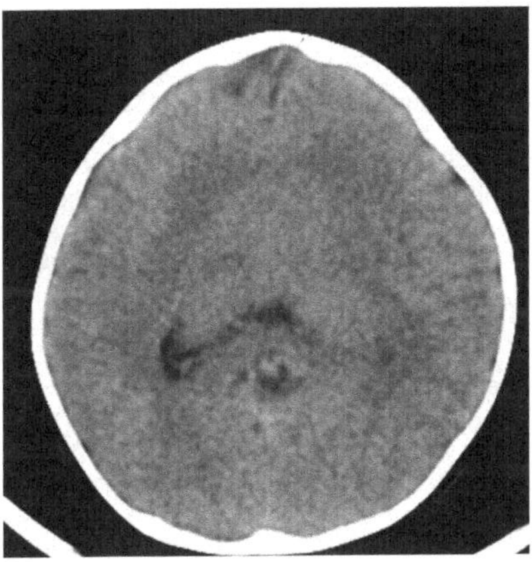

Figure 9.31

ANSWER KEYS

Figure 9.1: Axial NCCT head showing diffuse brain edema with effacement of sulcal spaces, ventricles and preserved attenuation of basal ganglia, thalami suggestive of 'reversal sign' in a case of hypoxic-ischemic brain injury.

Figure 9.2: Axial NCCT head showing diffuse brain edema with effacement of sulcal spaces, ventricles and preserved attenuation of cerebellar hemispheres suggestive of 'white cerebellum sign' in a case of hypoxic-ischemic brain injury.

Figure 9.3: Axial CT lung window sections showing consolidation in bilateral lungs suggestive of ARDS.

Figure 9.4: Axial CECT abdomen showing simple cysts studded in entire liver parenchyma in a case of polycystic liver disease.

Figure 9.5: Ultrasound image showing slightly hypoechoic liver and diffuse thickening of wall of gallbladder in a case of acute hepatitis.

Figure 9.6: CT scannogram head showing skull fracture with adjacent scalp hematoma.

Figure 9.7: Chest radiograph showing bilateral lucent hemithoraces with positive deep sulcus sign suggestive of bilateral pneumothorax.

Figure 9.8: Axial CECT abdomen showing heterogenously enhancing mass lesion in right kidney in a case of right Wilms' tumor.

Figure 9.9: Chest radiograph of a child showing cystic lesion in right upper zone suggestive of pneumatocele.

Figure 9.10: Radiograph of bilateral knee joints showing fraying and cupping of metaphyses suggestive of rickets.

Figure 9.11: Axial CECT abdomen images showing bowel loops in right thoracic cavity suggestive of congenital diaphragmatic hernia.

Figure 9.12: Axial contrast CT head showing ring enhancing lesions in brain parenchyma with disproportionate perilesional edema and midline shift in a case of multiple tuberculomas.

Figure 9.13: Intravenous urography film showing horseshoe kidney with bifid ureters on left side.

Figure 9.14: Axial CECT head showing extra-axial cystic lesion in right temporal fossa suggestive of arachnoid cyst.

Figure 9.15: Axial CECT head image showing bilateral basal ganglia calcification.

Figure 9.16: Coronal CECT abdomen showing thickening of ileocaecal region with adjacent necrotic lymph nodes suggestive of ileocaecal tuberculosis.

Figure 9.17: Axial CECT neck showing cystic lesion in relation to left parotid gland with hyperdense contents suggestive of Type I infected branchial cyst.

Figure 9.18: Axial CECT abdomen showing right psoas abscess with necrotic retroperitoneal lymph nodes suggestive of tubercular etiology.

Figure 9.19: Chest radiograph showing cystic lucencies in left hemithorax with ill-defined border of left hemidaphragm in a case of congenital diaphragmatic hernia.

Figure 9.20: Axial T2-weighted MR brain image showing cystic lesions scattered in brain parenchyma with eccentric scolex giving a 'starry sky appearance' in neurocysticercosis.

Figure 9.21: Axial NCCT head scan showing enlarged posterior fossa with cystic dilatation of fourth ventricle extending posteriorly in a case of Dandy-Walker syndrome associated with bilateral schizencephaly.

Figure 9.22: Axial CECT abdomen image showing horseshoe kidney with PUJO of left moiety.

Figure 9.23: Axial T1 contrast brain MR showing multiple ring enhancing lesions in brain parenchyma some of them appear conglomerated suggestive of tuberculomas.

Figure 9.24: X-ray skull lateral view showing lytic lesions in skull with no sclerosis in a case of histiocytosis.

Figure 9.25: Chest radiograph showing small millet sized nodules scattered in bilateral lung parenchyma in a case of miliary tuberculosis.

Figure 9.26: X-ray spine lateral view showing H-shaped vertebrae in a case of sickle cell disease.

Figure 9.27: Infantogram showing narrow thoracic cavity, short-tubular bones with a typical 'telephone handle' appearance in a case of thanatophoric dysplasia.

Figure 9.28: Chest radiograph showing boot shaped heart with pulmonary oligaemia in a case of Tetralogy of Fallot.

Figure 9.29: Skull X-ray lateral view showing copper beaten skull in a case of obstructive hydrocephalus.

Figure 9.30: Axial NCCT head showing subependymal calcified nodules in a case of tuberous sclerosis.

Figure 9.31: Axial NCCT head showing fused basal ganglia and thalami in case of lobar holoprosencephaly.

Index

R

S